Integrated Care in Action

of related interest

Creating Person-centred Organisations
Strategies and Tools for Managing Change in Health,
Social Care and the Voluntary Sector
Stephen Stirk and Helen Sanderson
ISBN 978 1 84905 260 3
eISBN 978 0 85700 549 6

The Individual Service Funds Handbook
Implementing Personal Budgets in Provider Organisations
Helen Sanderson and Robin Miller
ISBN 978 1 84905 423 2
eISBN 978 0 85700 792 6

Leading Good Care
The Task, Heart and Art of Managing Social Care
John Burton
Foreword by Debbie Sorkin
ISBN 978 1 84905 551 2
eISBN 978 0 85700 985 2

Emerging Values in Health Care
The Challenge for Professionals
Edited by Stephen Pattison, Ben Hannigan, Roisin Pill and Huw Thomas
ISBN 978 1 84310 947 1
eISBN 978 0 85700 365 2

How to Become a Better Manager in Social Work and Social Care
Essential Skills for Managing Care
Les Gallop and Trish Hafford-Letchfield
ISBN 978 1 84905 206 1
eISBN 978 0 85700 442 0

Whistleblowing and Ethics in Health and Social Care
Angie Ash
ISBN 978 1 84905 632 8
eISBN 978 1 78450 108 2

Integrated Care in Action

A PRACTICAL GUIDE FOR HEALTH, SOCIAL CARE AND HOUSING SUPPORT

Robin Miller, Hilary Brown and Catherine Mangan

Jessica Kingsley *Publishers*
London and Philadelphia

First published in 2016
by Jessica Kingsley Publishers
73 Collier Street
London N1 9BE, UK
and
400 Market Street, Suite 400
Philadelphia, PA 19106, USA

www.jkp.com

Library of Congress Cataloging in Publication Data
Names: Miller, Robin, 1968- author. | Brown, Hilary, 1949- author. | Mangan,
    Catherine, author.
Title: Integrated care in action : a practical guide for health, social care
    and housing support / Robin Miller, Hilary Brown and Catherine Mangan.
Description: Philadelphia : Jessica Kingsley Publishers, 2016. | Includes
    bibliographical references and index.
Identifiers: LCCN 2015049155 | ISBN 9781849056465 (alk. paper)
Subjects: LCSH: Social service. | Medical care. | Housing.
Classification: LCC HV40 .M527 2016 | DDC 361.0068--dc23 LC record available at
    http://lccn.loc.gov/2015049155

British Library Cataloguing in Publication Data
A CIP catalogue record for this book is available from the British Library

ISBN 978 1 84905 646 5
eISBN 978 1 78450 142 6

Printed and bound in Great Britain

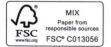

Contents

Acknowledgements

We would like to thank all those colleagues from the academic, practice and policy communities from whom we have drawn such inspiration and learning. Particular thanks must go to our reviewers, Kate Nixon and Steve Appleton, for reading a (very rough) first draft, and to Shamsul Rosunally, for patiently responding to our ever-changing amendments to the figures.

Preface

Integration of services is now a key aspiration within national and international policies in health, social care and supported housing. As a result, there is increasing expectation that managers, clinicians and practitioners within these services will be able to deliver integrated care on the ground. Most staff working in these sectors will understand and support the principles behind integration, as they will have undoubtedly experienced the frustrations of services being fragmented, and so delivering poor support and care. They will hopefully also have seen the benefits for patients, service users and their families when services are actually able to work together successfully. However, the best models through which these principles can be translated into practice and their individual contribution to such an integrated approach may not be so apparent. In part, this may be down to a lack of clarity about what integration is, due to the myriad of problems, services and needs that it is being connected with and the outcomes that it is supposed to deliver. Many will have been part of attempts to bring professionals and services together under previous policies connected with joint pathways, organisational partnerships or multi-disciplinary teams, to name a few, and may not be clear how current integration differs from these. Furthermore, earlier initiatives may not have worked as well as was hoped, or did deliver but were then subsequently disbanded due to a change in national priorities or local relationships. As a result, many people working in health, social care and supported housing may be confused, demoralised or feel daunted about being tasked with achieving integration.

Who is this handbook for?

This book seeks to address these uncertainties, frustrations and anxieties regarding integration through explaining what it means in practice, sharing lessons from what has worked elsewhere, and providing tools, techniques and approaches that can support the process of change. It is written primarily for those managers who will be tasked with achieving integrated care on the ground, and in particular those tasked with setting up a new *integrated care initiative*. The leaders of practice bridge the gap between the aspirational visions of national, local and organisational strategies and the realities of limited budgets, variable staffing and increasing demand. These leaders, and the roles that they play, are many – unit and service managers of rehabilitation and long-term support options for older people and people of working age with mental health problems, disability and/or frailty; senior practitioners and operational managers within community mental health teams, care management teams and hospital discharge teams; commissioners undertaking service redesign across complex pathways of health, housing and care; and doctors and other clinicians who have a key role in ensuring services are coordinated across a range of disciplines and professionals. Whilst in the past these practice leaders of integration were often employed within the NHS or local government, they are now also based within the voluntary and community sector and in some parts of the UK within private agencies. Increasingly integration is being seen as the 'norm' rather than as the 'exception'.

What is the approach taken?

It often appears that policy is describing 'integrated care' as a fixed way of working that must be achieved and, once established, is then set in stone. In this book, we take the view that integration is concerned with a fluid set of interactions between individuals accessing services and their families, the professionals and practitioners who support them, and the organisations and policy contexts that these staff work within. Many individuals access multiple services over the course of their lives, and require different professionals and services to work together in response to their needs and aspirations. Integration and integrated care are therefore never likely to be 'achieved' in full for all services and all the individuals who need to access them. As Leutz famously quoted, 'your integration is my fragmentation' – if they are achieved in one set of services, this may be at the cost of less integration with other services (Leutz 1999, p.91). Furthermore, they are unlikely to remain so for long, as key staff members move into new jobs, services and organisations become restructured, and policy directions and priorities are changed. These fluid circumstances require integrated care leaders to be engaged, informed, adaptive and responsive to the fluctuating demands, expectations and opportunities. That said, we know from previous research and practice experience that there are a set of key building blocks that need to be in place to enable an integrated care initiative to provide a solid foundation for improving the lives of people and their families. These building blocks cannot be established once and then left alone; rather, they will need constant tending and altering as others are created and circumstances change. The kaleidoscopic image on the front cover of this book reflects the opportunity to shape these building blocks and how they interact to provide different patterns and interpretations that depend on local circumstances and needs.

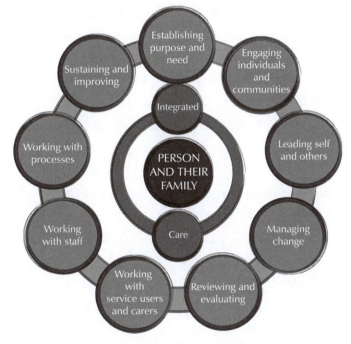

Figure 1: Building blocks of an integrated care initiative

In this book we consider the key building blocks of integration (see Figure 1 above). It should be noted that whilst for pragmatic purposes there is a need to have a starting point, they can't be tackled in a tidy linear sequence. Instead, the building blocks have to be addressed interactively, with previous blocks revisited and improved over time. There is also no one design of each building block that will work in each circumstance. Instead, we provide the learning about the key issues that should be considered, and present frameworks and models that will be helpful in the planning and delivery of integrated care initiatives. To help illustrate what these look like in practice, we draw on real *case examples* from previous and current initiatives. A set of *fictional scenarios* of integration based on common 'wicked issues' (see Chapter 1) are also explored to demonstrate how the building blocks could be approached in different contexts and to achieve alternative aims. Key organisations that can provide other resources on integrated care are provided at the end of the book.

What are the building blocks of integration?
Establishing purpose and need (Chapter 2)

- How can you find out what the issues are with the current arrangements?

- What are the outcomes you want to achieve?

- How can we map out the integrated care initiative?

- How can we be creative when designing an integrated initiative?

Engaging and involving individuals and communities (Chapter 3)

- Why do we engage and involve service users, carers and citizens?

- What activities do we engage and involve service users, carers and citizens in?

- What are the barriers to engaging and involving people in integrated initiatives?

- Which factors enable engagement and involvement?

- What are the key stages of involvement?

Leading self and others (Chapter 4)

- How can you lead change when you're not in charge?

- What is the environment in which you are leading and the task to be done?

- What are the frameworks to help the leading of change in a complex environment?
- How can you develop resilience for self, and for your team?

Managing change: processes and people (Chapter 5)

- How can we keep change on track?
- What approaches will build change for the future?
- Who are the key stakeholders and what is their influence?
- How can we positively support staff in the change process?
- What enables good communication?

Evaluating and reviewing integration (Chapter 6)

- What are the key issues before getting started on an evaluative review?
- What methods will help you to understand 'process' and 'benefits'?
- How can you learn from and share your findings?

Working with service users and carers (Chapter 7)

- What is the difference between self-efficacy, personal activation and advocacy?
- How can we support people to be 'self-caring' and 'self-managing'?
- What contribution can peer support networks make to integrated care?
- Is it possible to put people at the centre of decisions about their care?
- How can we design services in true partnership with service users?

Working with staff (Chapter 8)

- What are the common difficulties in professions working together?

- What are the skills, knowledge and values required for inter-professional working?

- How can we understand organisational culture?

- How can we use supervision within an integrated care initiative?

- What contribution can training and development make?

- How can we develop good team working?

- Can communities of practice make a positive contribution?

Working with processes and systems (Chapter 9)

- What systems and processes will support prioritisation of services across the population?

- What systems and processes will support coordination across organisations?

- What systems and processes will support sharing of data and information between professionals and between professionals and individuals?

- What systems and processes will support quality and probity?

Sustaining and improving (Chapter 10)

- What are the common reasons that an integrated care initiative can lose its way?

- What can be done to ensure that an initiative continues to improve and be sustained?

- How is it best to ensure that the end of an initiative is not the end of integrated care?

Key Terms

Carer Anyone either actively involved in the act of non-paid care-giving to an individual, or with a responsibility for the welfare of an individual, such as a parent or guardian.

Commissioning The process by which public services plan the services that are needed by the people who live in the local area, ensuring that services are available, high quality and appropriate. Commissioning is sometimes described as a cycle involving assessing the needs of the local population, deciding what services are needed, designing a strategy to deliver those services, making sure those services are in place, evaluating how well these services are working, and then making any changes needed. This is a broader process than simply choosing and paying a particular service provider to deliver a specific service on behalf of local people (a process often known as 'contracting' or 'procurement').

Integrated care This is achieved when a service user describes their care as follows: 'I can plan my care and support with people who work together to understand me and my carers, allow me control, and bring together services to achieve the outcomes important to me' (National Voices 2013).

Integrated care initiative A project or service that seeks to provide integrated care for individuals and their families by enabling better joint working across the relevant staff, teams, services and organisations in health, social care and housing support service.

Integration A process that seeks to create connectivity, alignment and collaboration within and between the cure, care and support sectors. It achieves this through addressing fragmentation in practice, management, funding and/or commissioning. The overall goals of integration are to improve the quality of life of individuals and their families, to increase the efficiency of resource usage, and to address health and societal inequalities (Berwick, Nolan and Whittington 2008; Kodner and Spreeuwenberg 2002).

Manager An individual employed to oversee and coordinate the financial, human and physical resources deployed by organisation(s) to achieve set objectives and responsibilities.

Outcome An aim or objective that people would like to achieve or need to happen, for example continuing to live at home, or being able to go out and about.

Person-centred planning A care-planning process that starts with the individual and what their needs and preferences are, and not with the services and what is available.

Practitioner An individual employed to directly provide housing support, social care or healthcare services to service users and carers who is not a member of a professional group but requires particular skills, knowledge and values. Examples include a tenancy support worker, a domiciliary care worker or nursing or therapy assistant.

Professional An individual who is accredited by a professional body to undertake a particular role following successful completion of a course of study and ongoing professional development. Examples include social worker, nurse, physiotherapist, psychologist and doctor.

Service user Someone actively in receipt of a health, social care or housing support service regardless of the nature of that service or their underlying needs.

System The interconnected organisations and services that have to work together to achieve integrated care for the population concerned.

Wicked issue A problem within society that is long-standing, complex and resistant to change.

Chapter 1

Integrated Care
An Introduction

As set out in the Preface to this book, at the heart of integrated care is a simple principle – that professionals and organisations who work with people with health, social care, housing support and other needs should collaborate around these individuals and their families to provide high quality care and treatment. This basic principle can be found within national policy, best practice guidelines and even within legislative duties in all of the home nations in the UK. It is also being promoted across Europe, North America and further afield with the World Health Organization (WHO) promoting a global strategy on person-centred and integrated care. As is so often the way, though, once we start to think what such an apparently simple principle means in practice, life becomes much more complicated and uncertain. What exactly is meant by 'integration' and 'integrated care'? Is it different to 'collaboration', 'joint working' and other such concepts? Who is being integrated and who is not? Are these latter services therefore fragmented? Which integrated care model works best?

To those responsible for developing integrated care initiatives on the ground, these might seem like academic debates. However, they do highlight key issues that need to be addressed if new processes, practices and partnerships are going to have a solid chance of succeeding. Furthermore, it is difficult for professionals and their organisations to provide integrated care if they have fundamentally different views of what integration is and what it can achieve. In this chapter we cover the themes below, and also introduce a set of 'wicked issues' (or problems) for which integration is often seen as the solution. These problems, and the integrated care initiatives that are developed to address them, are considered as we discuss the building blocks of integration.

- Why is integration being promoted in policy and practice?
- How can we understand integration?
- What is the evidence about what works in integrated care?

Why is integration being promoted in policy and practice?

Most people naturally see the potential benefits of professionals and their organisations working together, and indeed would assume that this would normally be the case in health, social care and housing support services. A key issue that quickly comes to mind is the importance of ensuring that there is necessary coordination and communication between professionals involved with particular individuals and their families, or that there is sufficient joint planning around what services are required in a locality to meet the needs of a defined population. These, however, are only part of the motivating factors that encourage (or not) organisations and the staff within them to actively participate in integration. Understanding these, and therefore the factors behind why an integrated care initiative may be suggested, can be a helpful context (and something that we explore in more detail next, in Chapter 2). The list below contains six common reasons why governments, partnerships and organisations look to integration:

- *To tackle so-called 'wicked issues':* Wicked issues are problems within society that are seen to be long-standing, complex and resistant to change. Examples include high levels of vandalism and crime in deprived neighbourhoods, increasing levels of obesity in young people and the connected health impacts, unemployment amongst people with mental health problems, and the sexual abuse of people with a learning disability (see Table 1.1 for the particular examples of wicked issues we follow during the book). It is thought that no single agency can respond to these wicked issues in isolation, partly because their resources are insufficient, but also because such problems require a more creative and holistic approach than such agencies have previously been able to deliver.

- *To ensure that individuals are protected from harm:* One wicked issue in particular to which integration has been associated is preventing children and vulnerable adults being abused. The problems of fragmentation in the current system have been identified within countless serious case reviews of the abuse of children and vulnerable adults, and it is therefore often hard not to become cynical about the often used comment that 'lessons will be learned' about the need for agencies to work better together. Integration is seen as essential to agencies identifying those at risk of being abused and so to providing proactive preventative support, picking up any concerns at an early point, and responding quickly and thoroughly to abuse that is identified. Integration has also been connected with ensuring that the quality of services in general is of a sufficient standard and abusive regimes are not allowed to develop or continue.

- *To improve people's outcomes and experience of accessing care:* Alongside the prevention of harm is increasing recognition that a key purpose of such services is to enable the people who access such support to have a better quality of life and to achieve their personal goals and aspirations. Failure by services to respond to their individual situations and needs may be because the separate services do not adequately listen to their requirements and experiences or have the necessary resources and skills to respond. These might be in place, however, but due to insufficient communication and cooperation between the agencies concerned, these are not translated into the desired outcomes. Linked to this issue is that of people's experience of accessing services. It is extremely frustrating for all concerned if the necessary information is not passed between agencies, or if someone is caught in an argument about resources and liability, which means that the support required is not provided.

- *To ensure that available resources are used efficiently:* The need to use available resources as efficiently as possible has also been a necessity for health, social care and housing agencies. As demands increase through changing demographics and public expectations whilst resources are at best stagnant and in some cases declining, there is more need than ever to ensure that any funding is used as well as is possible. Integration is seen as contributing to such greater efficiency in three main ways. First, it is recognised that the support provided can be duplicated across different agencies and integration should help to flush out such overlaps and ensure that it is only provided once. Second, support from one agency may need the involvement of another organisation to be successful, and if their offers are not coordinated, this may not be forthcoming at the correct time and in the correct format. Finally, due to a lack of joined-up planning, there may be an incorrect balance of different service options in a locality, meaning that more people than is necessary access expensive services on a long-term basis.

- *To meet a statutory requirement:* Alongside the general commitment that most agencies and individuals within them will have to work with their partners and colleagues, there are also central government mandates that require them to work together in certain circumstances. Therefore, even if they do not see this aspect of integration as being a current priority for their locality, they are expected to participate within the designated processes and activities. The nature of the demands can vary from a general requirement that they work with other agencies, to the coordination of a particular partnership forum. The type of mandate also varies, from a legal duty to a recommendation within good practice guidelines or strategy, and the arrangements regarding its implementation can influence the degree to which the integration in question will be prioritised. Legal duties (failure to meet them can lead to action through courts and financial compensation) and those with high profile performance monitoring processes will generally take precedence.

- *To enable organisational survival and growth:* Whilst perhaps less explicitly mentioned than many of the aspirations outlined above, there is no doubt that, for some organisations, integration is also a means to ensure that they are able to attract or at least maintain resources. This could be seen as a 'selfish' motivation to ensure their own survival and therefore the employment possibilities of their senior management and board, but it is generally also connected with a wish to continue with the services and staff that they have a belief in. Alongside financial and other physical resources there may also be an interest in maintaining local status and influence as accountability moves from traditional silos to more interconnected arrangements in which power is not as guaranteed and based on historical traditions.

How can we understand integration?

Integrated care will, of course, look different for each individual and their family due to their unique set of social circumstances, health conditions, local community and personal assets (see Table 1.1). Similarly, the services and functions that need to be part of an integrated care initiative will vary depending on the underlying problems and opportunities, expected outcomes, financial and other resources available, and level of commitment and interest of the key stakeholders. Our previous practical experience and the policy areas that we work within will shape what we understand as 'integrated care' and what 'integration' is required to achieve it in practice. Such learning and insights are as important and valid as those of someone with a different background. However, there is a danger that we fail to see the limitations of our knowledge, and that we miss opportunities to approach integration differently because we are too 'stuck in our ways'. There is also the potential that we are not able to communicate our thoughts and ideas clearly to people from a different sector who may have an alternative interpretation of key definitions or models.

Table 1.1: Examples of wicked issues and the people who have to survive within them

Wicked issue	The people who have to survive this wicked issue
Police are reporting increasing levels of low-level crime within the city centre. This is thought to be related to the number of homeless people who have complex needs related to mental illness and/or substance misuse	John is 30 years old and is homeless following his eviction from a hostel due to aggression to other tenants. He abuses alcohol, has severe mental health problems, and has spent time in prison. A local gang regularly steals his benefits
The finance team in the local authority is predicting that the learning disability placement budget will significantly overspend on out-of-borough placements for the third year in a row	Imran is 18 years old with severe learning and physical disabilities. He also has autism and can display challenging behaviour. He is due to leave school at the end of year. His mother would like to care for him but is struggling with his behaviour and physical size

cont.

Wicked issue	The people who have to survive this wicked issue
The acute hospital is reporting that there are increasing numbers of older people whose discharge from hospital is being delayed due to a lack of social care support, and that the A&E department is finding it difficult to cope with current demand	Patricia is 82 years old and lives in sheltered accommodation with her husband Leroy. He has dementia, and relies on Patricia to manage day-to-day tasks and to keep him safe. Patricia has been admitted to hospital following a stroke. Leroy has been staying in residential care whilst Patricia is an in-patient. She is physically ready for discharge but is not sure how she will cope when she returns home
A local women's group for Asian elders has noticed that the levels of depression appear to be rising. The area, which has a predominantly South Asian community, has high rates of type 2 diabetes	Balbir is 65 years old and is mother to three grown-up children. She has developed diabetes and found it difficult to control her diet and now has to inject insulin. She is very anxious about losing her sight and has had a leg ulcer following a fall at home

Note: Whilst fictional, these examples are based on real issues and real people.

One way of better understanding what we mean by integration and the key elements of the integrated care initiative that we are developing is to draw on 'conceptual' typologies. Four key frameworks are outlined below: the partnership map, micro to macro integration, vertical and horizontal integration, and processes of integration.

The partnership map

The partnership map (see Figure 1.1) displays the 'degree' or 'intensity' of integration (the 'depth') and the range of services involved in this integration (the 'breadth'). For example, a mental health partnership trust that has brought together specialist services for adults with mental health services would be described as 'deep' integration as the services are amalgamated within a single organisation, but if it only focuses on health and social care needs, it would not have a 'breadth' of services. A hospital discharge pathway that considers the role of different agencies in responding to the health needs, social care support and accommodation options is a looser form of integration, but has greater 'breadth' as it is also considering housing services. The wide range of community groups that provide education and leisure opportunities will usually have little formal connections other than being listed in a resource directory with contact details – this reflects little 'depth' but considerable 'breadth' of integration.

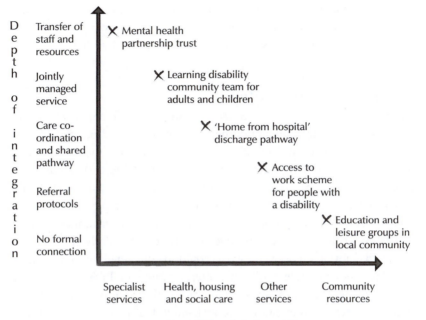

Figure 1.1: *The partnership map (based on Glasby 2005)*

The 'depth' of integration covers the following variables:

- *No formal connection* indicates that there is no particular integration agreement beyond the usual access and information processes in operation for these services.

- *Referral protocols* suggests that the agencies have agreed a particular process to request support from each other in relation to a particular population.

- *Shared pathway* suggests that the agencies have agreed not only how to refer to each other's service, but that they have agreed how they will respectively provide support during a particular stage of someone's illness or situation. This may include agreement about who will act as the nominated coordinator of the different inputs that someone receives.

- *Jointly managed* suggests that the staff from different agencies are working within the same service with one line management structure and agreed internal policies and procedures. This service may also have authority for delegated budgets from the services concerned.

- *Formal merger* suggests that staff and resources have been transferred to another organisation that is now accountable for their work and ensuring that their duties are fulfilled.

Micro to macro integration

Micro to macro concepts are used to suggest different levels within systems, and are used widely in the study of policy and practice. 'Micro' describes the smallest unit of operation and 'macro' the largest, with 'meso' essentially being the unit in between (see Table 1.2). Whilst these terms are commonly used to provide comparison between levels, the actual scale of these levels can be different. For example, 'macro' could mean a single organisation, partnership between organisations within a locality, or a national perspective of a system. Similarly there can be alternative interpretations of what could be included within units of operation. For example, whilst the interpretations in Table 1.2 are those commonly deployed in studies of integration, there are examples in which 'micro' is seen as integration amongst individual practitioners within a single organisation, 'meso' between practitioners working in different organisations, and 'macro' being organisation-to-organisation working (RAND Europe 2012).

Table 1.2: Micro to macro

Level	Interpretation	Example
Micro	Frontline clinicians and practitioners who have direct contact with the service user and their carer	The home care team, community psychiatric nurse, carer support worker and memory clinic that support an older person with dementia and their partner
Meso	Teams and services in relation to a targeted population	An assertive outreach team for people with severe mental health problems
Macro	Single organisations and whole system planning and coordination	Housing associations that provide care and support Integration Joint Boards in Scotland

Vertical and horizontal integration

Vertical integration is commonly used to refer to joint working between services that work with people as they progress through stages of their health or social crisis, recovery or condition. This will often be provided in alternative settings, require decreasing intensity of care and can be provided in a linear sequence (see Figure 1.2). Common examples would be a stroke rehabilitation pathway or a hospital avoidance protocol for people with mental health problems in crisis. *Horizontal* integration is commonly used to denote joint working between services working in parallel with someone at a similar stage in their crisis, recovery or condition, and within the same setting (often their own home).

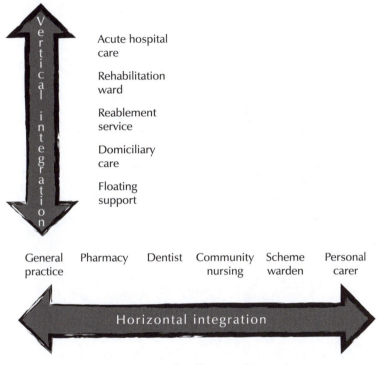

Figure 1.2: Vertical and horizontal integration

Processes of integration

Another way to think about what might be brought together in order to improve the integrated care experienced by service users is to consider the 'processes' that are involved. This includes processes that would involve frontline practitioners and clinicians, and also those that are more concerned with back office functions. The latter can contribute indirectly to integrated care through, for example, enabling more joined-up management of different professionals or the sharing of data on patient electronic records to avoid service users having to repeat the same information. Integration can therefore require involvement from a range of functions within the services and organisations concerned and a number of different mechanisms and approaches. These are represented in Figure 1.3, with more detail on the processes below.

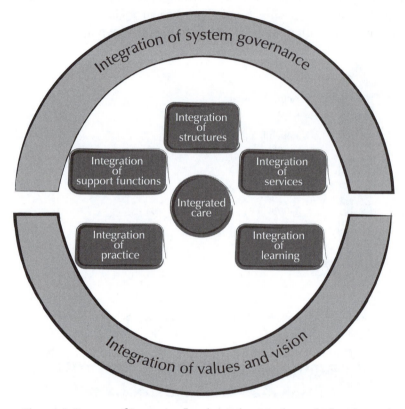

Figure 1.3: Processes of integration (based on Fulop, Mowlem and Edwards 2005)

- *Integration of structures:* organisations being merged together, the creation of a new organisation, contractual agreements between two or more organisations, joint planning bodies.

- *Integration of support functions:* one organisation taking on functions such as human resources (HR), finance, information technology (IT), procurement support on behalf of others, jointly outsourcing to another organisation.

- *Integration of services:* staff, funding and/or other resources are brought together from separate organisations into a single service that is jointly managed.

- *Integration of practice:* care pathways, shared guidelines and case management processes that connect the work of different professionals and services in the service user journey.

- *Integration of learning:* training and development opportunities that can be accessed by staff from different organisations and that can be jointly funded and delivered.

- *Integration of values and vision:* development of a common vision of what the separate organisations and services will achieve and the principles that will guide their work.

- *Integration of systems governance:* a coming together of the outcome frameworks, performance monitoring and incentives (both financial and reputational) through which separate organisations are held accountable.

What is the evidence about what works in integrated care?

Integrated care in its various guises has been the subject of considerable research over many years in the UK and internationally. Indeed, there are several academic journals dedicated to related articles along with countless others in housing, health and social care publications (see the Resources section at the end of this book). Despite all this attention, reviews of the available research consistently highlight that it is far from clear that integration always makes a difference or that it provides better care than non-integrated arrangements. Examples of the overall findings of such reviews are given in Box 1.1.

Along with highlighting weaknesses in the knowledge base, these also point to a number of potential factors that contribute to this lack of a convincing evidence base. These include the *quality* of research studies, and in particular, whether they are based on recognised and validated measures, considered 'counterfactual' (i.e. what would have happened in any case), and include the comparison with non-integrated arrangements; the *complexity* of evaluating a set of interacting elements that are also subject to other influences and context-specific changes; and a common *lack of focus* on benefits for service users rather than service efficiency and process. More fundamentally, there is an argument that it is not feasible to bring together such a diverse set of methods and approaches under the single banner of integration, and that integration is, in any case, an evolving process rather than a fixed arrangement.

Box 1.1: Key reviews of integrated care

Based on the evidence presented here, there may be a need to revisit our understanding of what integrated care is and what it seeks to achieve, and the extent to which the strategy lends itself to evaluation in a way that would allow for the generation of clear-cut evidence, given its polymorphous nature. (Nolte and Pitchforth 2014, p.vi)

The evidence base underpinning joint and integrated working remains less than compelling. It largely consists of small-scale evaluations of local initiatives which are often of poor quality and poorly reported. (Cameron et al. 2012, p.1)

Logic would require that engagement with the integration agenda is predicated on the assumption that it is a preferable alternative; moreover it would not seem unreasonable to presume that some form of integration is likely to be more effective in delivery than two or more agencies operating on their own. The available evidence base however suggests not only, inevitably, that the picture is complex, but that certain elements may be counter-intuitive. (Petch 2012, p.80)

…there is very little evidence that links the use of such services with what might be termed real and sustained outcomes for users: no demonstrable or measurable improvements in social or cognitive functioning, independence or quality of life. (Rummery 2009, p.1802)

At this point you may be wondering if it is worth all the effort to develop an integrated care initiative. Despite the limitations of the evidence, there are clear signs that integration of *appropriate services* for *some service users* can be of some benefit *in some circumstances* if they are *managed and supported appropriately*. Furthermore, there is a huge weight of evidence that fragmentation of services can lead to poor outcomes and efficiencies, and a lack of evidence that silo working is better than integrated working.

The main message to take from the evidence base is that integration will only work if done properly (another central belief of this book). The evidence also indicates that key enablers and barriers have been commonly found in integrated care initiatives (see Table 1.3). Often a barrier is the lack of an enabler and vice versa, and to avoid duplication, we have not listed these on the basis that you can simply reverse the positive findings.

There are also examples of research indicating that the same factor has been found to be an enabler in some circumstances and a barrier in others – for example, co-location of staff can provide an opportunity for informal contact and relationship building, but can also highlight differences in working conditions and lead to inter-professional rivalries.

Funding is usually an issue, both in relation to adequacy of resources to oversee and implement the change process and the potential for the double running of services whilst new models are introduced. It can also be a motivator, and sometimes a particularly daunting need for efficiency and savings can result in the most radical and innovative initiatives being developed.

Table 1.3: Enablers and barriers of integrated care from research

Element	Enablers	Barriers
Purpose of integration	Professionals and agencies understand the vision, aims and objectives Outcomes are specified and agreed by all stakeholders	Lack of shared understanding or agreement about purpose Competing visions about purpose and who is the lead agency Lack of robust and timely measurement of outcomes
Context	Previous positive history of joint working	Difficulties in staff recruitment and retention Constant reorganisation and lack of coterminosity
Leadership and management	Strong leadership at all levels and across organisational and professional boundaries Engaging people who access services in the planning and development Strong management and professional support	Lack of involvement of professionals in the design of the initiative Poor relationships between agencies and senior managers

cont.

Element	Enablers	Barriers
Practicalities	Realistic view as to the timescales required to achieve integrated care Adequate resources to support the development and launch of an initiative Co-location of staff from different professions and agencies	Co-location can lead to feelings of isolation from similar professionals
Staff and teams	Roles and responsibilities of staff are clear, and development provided to achieve these Teams have a clear purpose and are well managed	Unclear accountabilities for aspects of care or decisions
Culture and professions	Acknowledgement of the importance of culture and fostering of a new culture of collaboration Regular team meetings and team-building opportunities Appreciation of the contexts and pressures that other professionals and agencies work under	Negative views and stereotypes of other professions and agencies Different professional cultures and philosophies Lack of trust in other professionals' skills and judgements Status issues and hierarchical conflict between professionals
Communication	Effective communication and information sharing Adequate IT systems	Poor communication across organisational boundaries Practical difficulties and/or professional reluctance to share information
Finance	Explicit agreement about financial contributions, pooling of budgets and risk management	Uncertainty in funding for initiative or wider organisations Payment systems based on silo working and do not incentivise integrated care

Sources: Atkinson, Jones and Lamont (2007); Cameron et al. (2012); Frontier Economics (2012); Glasby et al. (2013); Miller (2013); Petch (2012)

Chapter 2

Establishing Purpose and Need

Chapter 1 set out some general aims of integration, but when considering an integrated care initiative, you need to understand why you are doing it in order to create an effective, tailored approach that addresses the particular issues in your area. Are you trying to integrate because the current system is broken and failing your users and carers, or are you trying to improve your current approach or improve the outcomes people are achieving, or a mix of all three? One of the problems for those seeking to implement integration is that there isn't a clear evidence base about what works, or which initiatives will best deliver improved outcomes. This means that there is no blueprint for those seeking to implement integration, and that each locality or service will need to develop an approach that meets the needs for people in their area and the context in which they are working. It is tempting to believe that if we implement x, then y will happen, but in a complex system that involves people, professionals and politicians, there is very rarely a simple solution that will deliver expected results.

So this chapter doesn't seek to tell you what or how to integrate, but offers you some useful questions to ask yourself as you develop your new approach, including:

- How can you find out what the issues are with the current arrangements?

- What are the outcomes you want to achieve?

- How can you map out the integrated care initiative?

- How can you be creative when designing an integrated initiative?

How can you find out what the issues are with the current arrangements?

In Chapter 1 four 'wicked issues' were set out that are typical of local situations that lead to the development of an integrated care initiative. Faced with the political, financial and personal pressures that commonly build around such situations, it is easy for services to jump to a solution before fully understanding the issues that lie behind them. Whilst there is always a chance that this could be just the right solution for the problem concerned, it is likely that this will not be the case. It is therefore vital that time is spent in understanding 'what works' and 'what doesn't' before recommending how best to respond. Table 2.1 shows how the wicked issues introduced in Chapter 1 could be explored, with more detail in the remainder of this section on these sources of data, tools and approaches that can be used to understand this data.

Data sources

Understanding user pathways and journeys: Developing stories of how people experience services in their current state is a powerful way of describing the system and understanding its impact on individuals. Several areas created fictional 'typical' users of services to help them understand gaps and duplication in the system and to identify the impact of any changes on individuals. For example, in Liverpool they created 'Our Ted', and in Cumbria they used the fictional 'Mrs Carlisle'. The North Wales Regional Single Point of Access Programme adapted the 'Mrs Smith' approach developed in Torbay to create postcards that could have been sent between friends to create the vision for what users want, and also to provide information for stakeholders about what the future could look like (see Figure 2.1). Journey mapping is a powerful way of telling the story of people who use our services, and can be done with users and carers and in multi-disciplinary teams, which helps people within the system to understand the issues, and may create an agenda for change. Involving users and their families in this, and working with them to design a more integrated, seamless and comprehensive pathway, is an excellent way of co-producing an integrated approach. All too often we forget that patients, users and carers are the experts in their own condition; they understand the impact that it has on their daily life – most importantly how they live with it outside the world of health, social care and housing – and can contribute hugely to improving their care and support pathways.

Table 2.1: Wicked issues and how the issues beneath them could be explored

Wicked issue	Could be explored by...
Homelessness	Understanding the user journey – work with homeless people already in receipt of services to carry out pathway mapping to understand their experiences, which services they interact with, and what support would help them
	Carrying out an audit of case files from across different agencies to understand the issues being faced by the services and the factors behind decisions
	Developing a multiple cause diagram to understand the factors involved in people becoming multiply excluded, and the links between them
	Analysing complaints data from the police about crime levels
	Using networks to identify best practice
A&E admissions	Developing a Pareto diagram (see page 36) to understand the factors at play and the impact they have to identify where to focus resources
	Developing a cause and effect diagram to understand why increasing numbers of older people are presenting to A&E
	Undertaking user pathway mapping to gain an understanding of the causes of entry to hospital and readmission
Diabetes	Consulting with older people from the South Asian community, using an advocacy group to understand levels of awareness of the causes of type 2 diabetes
	Undertaking user pathway mapping of a sample of 30 patients from the point of diagnosis
	Developing a cause and effect diagram based on the user pathway work
	Asking the neighbouring clinical commissioning group (CCG) with a similar population but lower rates of type 2 diabetes to conduct a three-day peer review of the service, in return for a reciprocal peer review in an area where they were performing better
Transition	Consulting with special schools, parents and young people to understand the needs of the individuals and to identify concerns and expectations for when they leave school
	Working with staff from across agencies to develop value stream mapping of the current learning disability service to understand the demands on and capacity of the team
	Using the 'five whys' to understand why young people were being placed out of area
	Carrying out an audit of recent case files to understand the reason behind decisions to place young people in out-of-area residential care

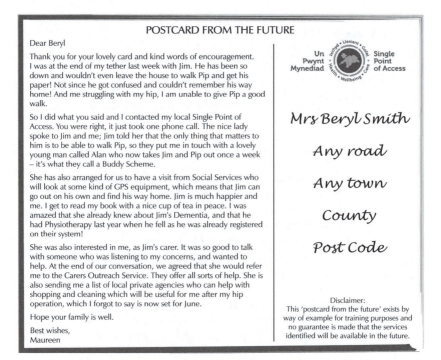

Figure 2.1: North Wales Regional Single Point of Access Programme

Rich pictures: Rich pictures can be used to illustrate complicated situations or issues, to help analyse a situation. They can be drawings, pictures, symbols or text that represent a particular situation or issue from the viewpoint of the people drawing them. They can show relationships, connections, influences and cause and effect, but also more subjective elements such as character and characteristics, as well as points of view, assumptions, etc. Rich pictures can be helpful in communicating issues between groups of people from different backgrounds and organisations where there may be cultural or language differences. Drawings, pictures and text can provide the basis for the shared understanding needed to enable further dialogue. People don't need to be able to draw, though – they can use stickers or cut out pictures from magazines, anything that is creative and reflects how they see the situation.

Audit of case notes and files: Case notes can provide an insight into the system and, in particular, where parts of the system are not working together effectively. You could review recent decisions that have been made about referrals, take a sample, or look at those where there was disagreement around the best outcome. Sharing these with other practitioners may provide interesting insights into the way in which professionals work together and how decisions are taken. From these insights you may be able to start to develop ideas about pathways and where agencies could better work together, to inform a more preventative, integrated pathway.

Analysing complaints data: Using anecdotal as well as more formal complaints data can be a rich source of data about what might be going wrong with current arrangements. For example, if staff members mention that a user has complained about being visited by lots of different people, or never seeing the same person twice, this is all data, and may be an indication of an inefficient system where there is duplication.

Survey feedback: There is likely to be a wealth of information about services as part of user surveys. The questions may not be exactly focused on issues that might be addressed through integration, but they are likely to be rich sources of data, especially open comments. Be curious and open about the data, and analyse it to see where gaps in quality of services lie.

Feedback from staff: Frontline teams are often those experiencing the sharp end of a fragmented system. Working with them to understand how the issues affect their work and the people they deal with can be a very powerful way of understanding how the approach is impacting on users and patients. For example, what is their experience of making referrals to other services? Do they receive feedback on what has happened to the referral? How do other professionals respond to them when they try and contact them to discuss an individual?

Direct consultation with service users and their carers and families: It may be that you do not have enough insight or evidence into your service and want to commission some primary research with people using your services. There are a range of different approaches (see Chapter 3) to support engagement with service users and their carers and families.

Peer review: Opening your service up to peer review can be a very powerful approach to getting an external, objective take on what's working well. You don't have to engage in a formal peer review approach – you could ask colleagues from other services to take part, or from a neighbouring area. They may want to use some of the approaches outlined above, such as interviewing users, creating pathways and looking at case files.

Understanding how to compare against benchmarks and best practice: What do you know about what best practice is and how your service compares? How does the performance of your service compare with others? A good way of understanding this is to visit other services that are willing to tell you about their experiences, and not always the best practice ones – there is a huge amount to learn from things that have not worked so well, as well as those areas that are highlighted as best practice.

Specific tools and methodologies

There is a wealth of change and organisational development tools that you can use to understand the current state. The Social Care Change Compendium (Miller *et al.* 2015) offers some helpful ideas. Here we have selected some of the most useful, and simple to use, approaches:

Multiple cause diagrams: This technique uses a picture to plot the relationships between parts of the system and to understand how different parts impact on others (see Figure 2.2). Various causes of a certain event or situation are represented, and relationships between variables in a given situation are investigated. Multiple cause diagrams explore why something has happened (often why something went wrong) or why a situation is as it is (often why a problem recurs). The multiple cause and effect diagram below illustrates the various causes for older people entering residential care, and the links between those.

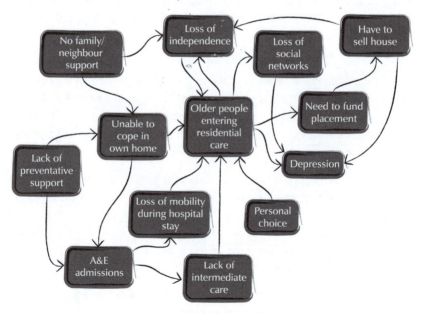

Figure 2.2: Multiple cause diagram

Cause and effect diagrams (also called 'fish bones'): A variation on the multiple cause approach above, this exercise is usually done with a team of those involved with the issue. The process starts with a 'why' – for example, 'Why do more people enter residential care earlier in our area than average?' Or 'Why are waiting times in hospital so long?' Potential causes are then mapped under specific headings, such as 'Materials', 'Methods', 'Equipment', 'Environment' and 'People', and links between the causes identified. The benefit of this approach is that it helps teams understand that there are many causes that contribute to an effect, it graphically displays the relationship of the causes to the effect and to each other, and it helps to identify areas for improvement. Figure 2.3 looks at the causes of provision of adaptations taking too long.

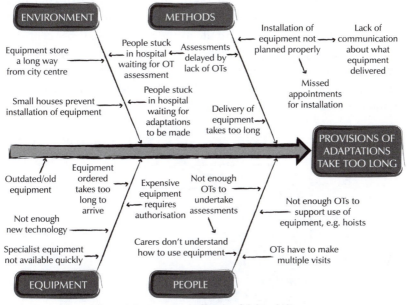

Figure 2.3: Cause and effect (or fish bone) diagram

Value stream mapping: This is part of 'lean' methodology, and can be particularly helpful in understanding what processes might not be working most effectively. The approach can be most usefully carried out with a multi-disciplinary team. The process requires mapping of all processes involved in providing a service – for example, all stages involved in the provision of adaptations to assist home living to identify value-giving and wasteful steps in the pathway. Start and end points are agreed – for example, diagnosis of a physical disability through to the provision of an aid. Those who come into contact with the client throughout the process undertake the mapping activity, initially looking at current practice on their own part of the pathway, and subsequently coming together to identify wasteful steps. From this you can produce a current state, and hence from there, an ideal state.

Pareto analysis: This is a type of chart that helps to identify the key issues that cause negative or positive impacts on a service. The technique helps you to focus efforts on the problems that offer the greatest potential for improvement. The chart is based on Pareto's principle (the 80/20 rule, that most things are not evenly distributed, and so, for example, 80 per cent of complaints are about 20 per cent of services, or 80 per cent of a nurse's time is spent on 20 per cent of patients). The number and/or percentage of different factors are mapped on a graph and put in order of frequency, with the most common on the left. Those that contribute to the first 80 per cent of an impact are seen as the most important ('the vital few'), with those that contribute to the remaining 20 per cent seen as relatively unimportant ('the trivial many'). It can be a helpful means to focus on the issues of most importance and so define how best to channel the available energy and resources. Figure 2.4 illustrates the data about complaints received about a care service.

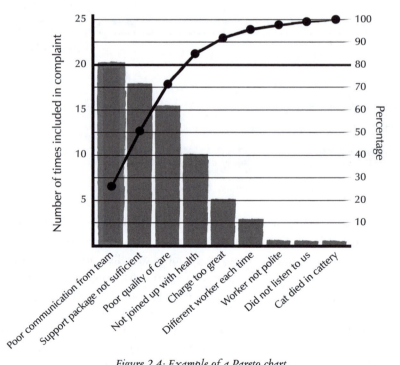

Figure 2.4: Example of a Pareto chart

Five whys: This approach is useful to guide the investigation of single problems or issues rather than explore an organisation holistically. A simple yet powerful approach, it enables the factors that lead to a situation to be identified through asking a series of questions related to the event or issue. Once a problem has occurred, the first 'why' question is 'Why did this happen?' It is likely that a number of answers will be found, and for each, the next 'why?' is asked: 'Why is that?' The sequence continues until the question has been asked and answered five times (see Table 2.2).

Table 2.2: Five whys

1. Why (did this happen)?	The young person with learning disabilities was placed in an out-of-area school	
2. Why (is that)?	There were no appropriate places available in the area	
3. Why (is that)?	The number of children with learning disabilities has risen	Schools have not been able to expand to increase capacity
4. Why (is that)?	High numbers of families have recently moved into the area	School sites are unsuitable for expansion
5. Why (is that)?	A large number of housing estates have recently been built, but with no additional school provision	Mainstream schools have not been willing to establish learning disability (LD) units on their sites

What are the outcomes you want to achieve?

As Chapter 1 suggests, there are often high-level, strategic aims of integration, to:

- tackle so-called 'wicked issues'
- ensure that individuals are protected from harm
- improve people's outcomes and experience of accessing care
- ensure that available resources are used efficiently
- meet a statutory requirement
- enable organisational survival and growth.

You may have some of these drivers for your integrated care initiative, and there may be a whole organisation mandate to integrate services. However, as someone who is going to develop a specific service or project, you need to develop a clear set of outcomes that you want to achieve.

One way of conceptualising these outcomes is through the 'triple aims' of integration (see Figures 2.5 and 2.6) (Berwick *et al.* 2008):

- raising the overall health of the community and addressing health inequalities (population health)

- improving people's experiences of care and their personal wellbeing (experience of care) *and*

- achieving more efficient use of resources through increased productivity and less intensive models of care (cost per head).

To achieve successful integration, all three of these aims are important, and it is short-sighted to achieve only one or two of them.

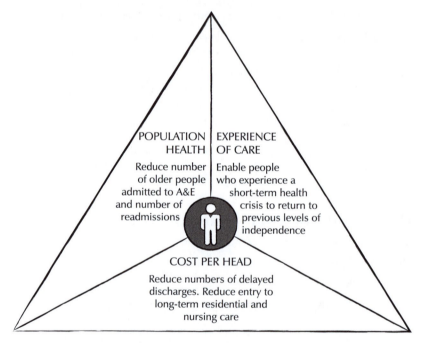

Figure 2.5: Triple aims in respect of the A&E admission scenario

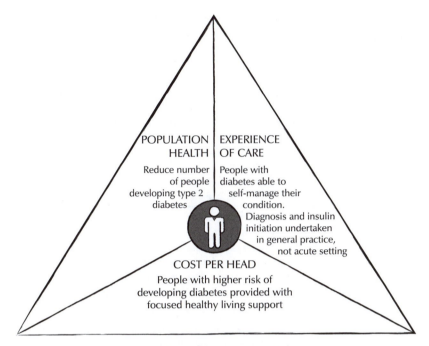

Figure 2.6: Triple aims in respect of the diabetes scenario

These aims can be viewed both at the macro level (whole population) and micro level (individuals). So, for example, the overarching aim of integration in your area might be about enabling people to remain in their homes for longer, and ensuring services are developed around individuals. You will want to think about how those aims play out for those individuals experiencing your services (micro level); for example, ensuring your service users do not need to repeat their stories over and over, can avoid unnecessary hospital admissions, have friends or neighbours who will pop in to support them, or that they are able to walk down to the local shops. It is essential to involve users and carers in discussions about what they want from your services, and it is useful to have both the macro and micro aspects in mind when developing an integrated approach. You may also want to include outcomes for professionals, such as job satisfaction, professional relationships, training and development.

The work that you have done to identify the issues within your current arrangements and to understand the way in which people experience your service will help inform the aims and outcomes that you want to achieve from your integrated initiative. These can be very specific to the service that you provide (see Table 2.3).

Table 2.3: Desired outcomes for the four wicked issues

Wicked issue	Desired outcomes
Homelessness	• For these individuals to have somewhere safe and warm to live and to have regular meals • For these individuals to access general healthcare and welfare benefits • For these individuals to get support in relation to dependency and mental health • To reduce perceived and actual increased levels of crime within the local community • To reduce the number of emergency admissions of multiply excluded homeless people
A&E admissions	• To enable people who experienced a short-term health or social crisis to return to their previous level of independence • To slow the rate of deterioration in the physical and mental health of people with long-term conditions • To reduce the use of A&E and readmissions to hospital • To reduce entry to long-term residential and nursing care • To maintain (reduce) numbers of delayed discharges
Diabetes	• To improve general awareness of the local community regarding the risk of diabetes through lifestyle and diet • To target those at higher risk of developing diabetes with focused healthy living support • To undertake diagnosis and if necessary insulin initiation in general practice rather than in the acute setting • To encourage those with diabetes to self-manage their condition and to avoid worsening and complications
Transition	• To carry on developing the young people's communication and independent living skills • To ensure the young people can maintain their key friendships from school • To ensure that parents/carers have the practical support that they need to continue to be the main carers • For the young people to continue to receive specialist health support when they transfer to adult services • For health and social care funding to be used efficiently and to develop local capacity and skills

How can we map out the integrated care initiative?

Having understood the strengths and weaknesses of the current situation and agreed on the outcomes to be achieved, it is now possible to think through how best to deliver these in practice. A key approach that will help you to identify outcomes and design and test your integrated initiative is to create a *theory of change*, or *logic*, model. These terms may sound confusing, but their approach provides a simple framework through which we can map out the various elements of an initiative, and how we think they will interact to provide the expected outcomes and impacts.

There are different schools of thought regarding the best way to map out and present the theory or logic of an intervention, and whilst these share common principles, they can vary in their use of terminology and what is emphasised in their mapping (see the Resources section at the end of this book). What is of particular debate is the issue of what an *outcome* and an *impact* is. We suggest five key elements that we have found helpful in unpicking integrated care initiatives that we combine under the term 'mapping': context, resources, activities, benefits and assumptions (see Figure 2.7).

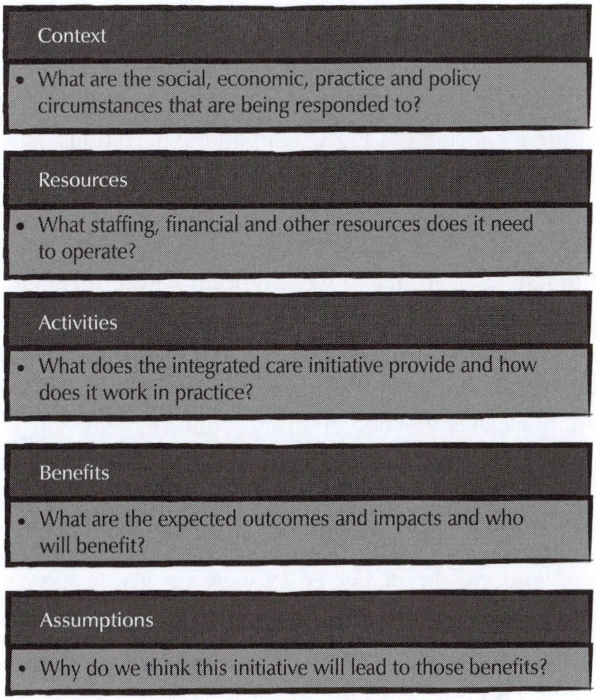

Context
- What are the social, economic, practice and policy circumstances that are being responded to?

Resources
- What staffing, financial and other resources does it need to operate?

Activities
- What does the integrated care initiative provide and how does it work in practice?

Benefits
- What are the expected outcomes and impacts and who will benefit?

Assumptions
- Why do we think this initiative will lead to those benefits?

Figure 2.7: Five key mapping elements

Context

There is increasing recognition of the importance of context in understanding how an integrated care initiative works and the benefits that it achieves. This is particularly important in terms of learning from different approaches. A project that has been successfully run in one area of a country may not be so successful in a different locality, and a new model trialled by a pilot project may not then deliver such good results when it is adopted in services. Talking through the context with your stakeholders is also important for the initiative itself, as it can provide a more complete view of what led to its development. Key aspects of context that we would suggest are included are as follows:

- local history of integrated care in this service area – what has been tried before?

- current strengths and weaknesses of local services (including the experiences of people who have accessed the service)

- current and future national policy context

- future local changes in demand and expectations.

Resources

You need to have a clear idea of what type and level of resources you will need to implement the initiative. This should encompass those that have been provided specifically for the service or project, and also existing resources that are required for its development and running. Even if the economic aspects are not of prime concern, you will still need to get a good overview of all the people, funds and technologies that will potentially contribute to the integration to understand how they connect and interact. Key resources that you may want to include are:

- *staff* who will be dedicated to working in the service, including managers and professional supervisors

- *budgets* that are available to the service in respect of both purchasing care and support for the service user and maintaining the service

- *equipment* that will be made available to service users to support their independence and wellbeing

- *technologies and systems* that will support the inter-professional working and delivery of integrated care

- *buildings* that will be used to provide support or to host the staff within the initiative

- *external partners* that the service will need to engage in its work, even if their resources remain separate.

Activities

The activities are the actions through which the identified resources will be connected together in order to provide the expected outcomes and impacts. There are a variety of potential activities that could be included, such as those that primarily operate within the service, for example a multi-disciplinary referral meeting or professional supervision processes, and those with an outward focus, such as care planning with service users or partnership meetings with other agencies.

The examples outlined in Case example 2.1 set out how a range of approaches involving a variety of agencies are likely to be needed to achieve the outcomes sought.

Case example 2.1: Developing integrated care initiatives

Integrated care initiative in Lincolnshire

In Lincolnshire, the outcome they wanted to achieve was for people with long-term conditions to remain in their own homes for as long as possible. To achieve this they established an integrated wellbeing service that supports proactive care. The approach includes:

» support to gain home management and lifestyle skills

» access to befriending services

» supporting access to various activities provided by local clubs and voluntary or community organisations

» support where people require help and advice to remain in their home

» support to secure and maintain appropriate housing

» help to manage finances and benefit claims

» help to complete forms to enable people to stay independent in their own homes

» support to understand the options available by gathering information and explaining it in a way that makes sense to people.

Integrated care initiative in Hertfordshire

Hertfordshire had some key outcomes they wanted to achieve through developing integrated services. These were to:

» support people to live independently at home to reduce unnecessary hospital or social care admissions

» improve the coordination of services around the needs of the person

» prevent unnecessary hospital admissions by offering alternative care in the community.

Hertfordshire developed a range of services to achieve these outcomes, for example *HomeFirst*, an integrated community support service that provides effective care for people at risk of hospital admission or social care placement. It brings together expertise from NHS and social care services to ensure service users get the right care and support to stay at home wherever possible. HomeFirst teams include nurses, occupational therapists (OTs), social workers and care staff. The service consists of two elements:

» a reactive rapid response service, where health and social care staff respond within 60 minutes to people in crisis

» a proactive virtual ward that supports people who are at risk of hospital admission; this helps keep people in their own home.

There is also the *Community Bed Bureau Scheme* that focuses on improving the management and coordination of community bed rehabilitation services. It coordinates, tracks and monitors the use of community beds, and assigns the person to a bed that most suits their needs. There are two main types of community beds:

» intermediate care, where need is mainly medical, usually to help a person recover from a period of ill health

» enablement, where a person is supported to regain their abilities and confidence to continue living independently.

What do these examples tell us?

» The outcomes that we often want to achieve from an integrated initiative are complex and varied.

» The interventions that are designed to achieve those outcomes will involve a wide range of specialist and universal services, partners and direct support, as well as preventative approaches.

Benefits

The expected benefits of the integrated care initiative should reflect the work done to develop the outcomes that you want to achieve from the integration. It is important that all stakeholders that were involved in the development and delivery of the integrated initiative have the same understanding of why the initiative is being put in place and what benefits they expect to achieve.

Assumptions

Assumptions are the 'theory' aspect of the mapping process in that they set out the 'beliefs' that we hold about the integrated care initiative, and why we think this combination of resources and activities will lead to the expected benefits. It is very common that these are not properly aired in the development of an initiative beyond the superficial level of 'integration is a good thing'. This is a potential problem, as it may be that stakeholders have different views of what they think will be the key to success, or the overall model is not correctly configured or sufficiently resourced to work in this context. Encouraging stakeholders to express these can lead to some difficult but necessary discussions about their alternative perspectives. The thinking about why the initiative will work can be done on the basis of the knowledge and insights that the stakeholders bring, but can also be informed from learning from similar initiatives seeking to bring about such benefits in comparable situations.

When undertaking the mapping and potential solutions, it is also important to remember that a new integrated care initiative is not necessarily a solution to every problem. In some cases a less radical solution may be equally as effective in addressing the problem. It's all about understanding what the issue is, what outcomes you want to achieve, and designing something that is likely to achieve them. The scenario presented in Table 2.4 suggests how an alternative solution might be reached.

Figure 2.8 provides an example of a mapping model in relation to the diabetes wicked issue scenario outlined in Chapter 1.

Table 2.4: Wicked issue in which a new integrated care initiative is not seen as the best solution

How did they design an integrated intervention to deliver these outcomes?
• Held an Open Space event for schools, parents, young people and health and learning disability teams to identify what could be achieved • Used the de Bono 'Six Thinking Hats' approach to develop the ideas raised at the Open Space event • Developed a theory of change model to understand the current system and what a different system might look like
What did the integrated initiative look like?
• Due to the very different needs and interests of the individuals and a move to access community resources rather than rely on segregated services, it was decided *not* to develop a new integrated care initiative • Instead, existing care planning processes across children and adult services will be improved, with additional funding for advocacy and person-centred planning services

How can we be creative when designing an integrated initiative?

A myriad of different approaches can be helpful when trying to think through options for achieving integrated care. We set out here some of the ones that we find most helpful in the context of integrated care and that are achievable without any external support.

Safe-fail experiments

Safe-fail experiments enable you to create a hypothesis, a safe opportunity to try it out, expand it if it works and close it down if it doesn't. This type of experimentation can be helpful when working within a complex system as there are unlikely to be repeating relationships between cause and effect, and small interventions may have a significant impact on how the system works, which cannot be predicted. They are small-scale, and approach issues from different angles, in order to reveal possible successful approaches.

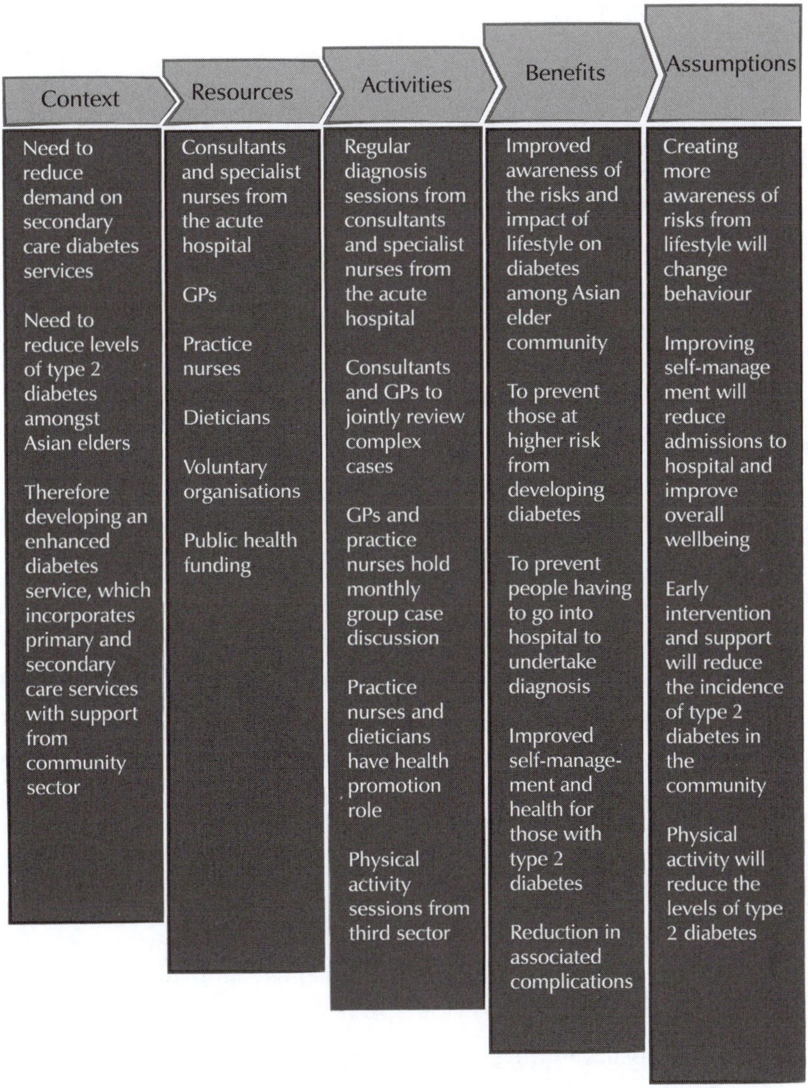

Context	Resources	Activities	Benefits	Assumptions
Need to reduce demand on secondary care diabetes services	Consultants and specialist nurses from the acute hospital	Regular diagnosis sessions from consultants and specialist nurses from the acute hospital	Improved awareness of the risks and impact of lifestyle on diabetes among Asian elder community	Creating more awareness of risks from lifestyle will change behaviour
Need to reduce levels of type 2 diabetes amongst Asian elders	GPs	Consultants and GPs to jointly review complex cases	To prevent those at higher risk from developing diabetes	Improving self-manage ment will reduce admissions to hospital and improve overall wellbeing
Therefore developing an enhanced diabetes service, which incorporates primary and secondary care services with support from community sector	Practice nurses	GPs and practice nurses hold monthly group case discussion	To prevent people having to go into hospital to undertake diagnosis	Early intervention and support will reduce the incidence of type 2 diabetes in the community
	Dieticians	Practice nurses and dieticians have health promotion role	Improved self-manage-ment and health for those with type 2 diabetes	Physical activity will reduce the levels of type 2 diabetes
	Voluntary organisations	Physical activity sessions from third sector	Reduction in associated complications	
	Public health funding			

Figure 2.8: Example of a mapping model

Key principles on how to manage a safe-fail experiment include the following (Leadership for Change 2013):

- *Experiment freely and expect failure:* Recognise that failure is good and promotes learning.

- *Consider as many ideas as possible for experimentation:* Any idea that has a remote possibility of creating an improvement that can be carried out within the next eight weeks.

- *Start with experiments where failure can be tolerated:* Choose experiments where the overall impact of failure on the system is likely to be small and/or manageable.

- *Be comfortable with 'safe uncertainty':* Provide just enough structure, just enough control and just enough planning to mitigate the biggest of risks whilst leaving enough fluidity, spontaneity and freedom to welcome new possibilities.

- *Design experiments that can be monitored:* To plan future experiments, you need to be able to determine whether the outcome of an experiment was favourable.

- *Run multiple experiments in parallel:* Over time, experiments producing undesirable results should be wound up and new experiments started in promising areas.

- *Share the results of your experiments with others, and learn from the results of their experiments:* But be wary that the complexity of systems and contexts means that results can be hard to replicate across different areas.

Asking powerful questions

A powerful way of thinking what type of integrated initiative you need to design is to ask yourself a series of 'powerful questions', such as:

- What issues in the system are adaptive challenges, and what are technical problems?

- Are there any of our projects or activities that we are treating as day-to-day management when they are really transformative change? (See Chapter 4 for more details.)

- What day-to-day management processes do we need?

- What connections do we need to make, what relationships to build? Are the right people involved?

- Are any power differentials stopping change?

- What is 'messy' that we need to live with? Are there opportunities for experiments? How can you help contain any anxiety (including yours)?

- Do you understand the rules that guide how the system works? (Even in complexity, there are often simple rules that lead to outcomes – for example, in the case of integration, the rules might be that, if in doubt, refer to hospital, always defer to senior consultants and give acute physical services priority over chronic and mental health. If these simple rules always determine what happens in the system, any integration effort needs to address these.)

Open Space approach

Open Space brings together groups of people to identify and address issues connected with a shared matter of interest. Its basis is that shared understanding built through participation will yield coordinated action. Its purpose is to surface differences in understanding, to work through them, and build a new response. Successful events require a compelling theme, attendance of all those with a stake in change, and relevant tasks to complete within subgroups during the event.

Open Space uses a minimal formal structure, allowing participants to self-organise around topics associated with the overarching conference theme. It is often beneficial to get an external facilitator who has used the Open Space methodology in order to get the best out of these events.

Appreciative Inquiry (AI)

Most approaches to change begin with identifying the 'problem' to be solved and working back to understand the causes of the problem, and therefore how it can be addressed. In contrast, AI frames change as a 'mystery' to be embraced, and starts from identifying the best of what could be, discussing what should be, and innovating what will be. It is sustained by the belief that social systems evolve in the direction of the positive images that individuals hold about them – looking forward and extending 'that which is going right'. The approach applies positive questions with the aim of surfacing, and then extending, 'positive core' ideas across the networks of individuals that make up organisations (see Figure 2.9).

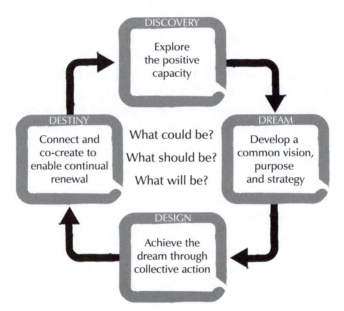

Figure 2.9: Appreciative Inquiry

De Bono's Six Thinking Hats[1]

The 'creative thinking' approach is a tool for stimulating focused group discussion, built on the assumption that the human brain may respond to challenges in six distinctive ways:

- information (white hat) – the facts at hand
- emotions (red hat) – intuitive reactions of emotional feeling
- discernment (black hat) – logic of caution
- optimism (yellow hat) – logic of possible benefits
- creativity (green hat) – investigation of possibilities
- meta thinking (blue hat) – a combination of the other types.

---

1   See www.debonogroup.com/six_thinking_hats.php

Each of these responses may be harnessed to encourage reflection on a specific problem/challenge/question. By organising participants to consider the problem specifically from each of the six perspectives, the group will be more creative in their response to the problem. The metaphor of 'six thinking hats' is adopted to describe the ordered use of the six approaches in the above sequence.

Below we bring the processes together to show how new integrated care initiatives were developed for three of our wicked issues (see Table 2.5).

Table 2.5: Responses to the wicked issue scenarios

High numbers of homeless people in the city are not able to live in the usual homeless accommodation
There is an increase in the number of multiply excluded homeless people in the city – those who commonly suffer from mental health problems, abuse alcohol/illegal substances and/or have contact with the criminal justice system (either as perpetrators or as victims). This population are not able to live in the usual homeless accommodation due to the chaotic nature of their lifestyles and/or because they have been banned due to use of drugs and/or violence.
How would you find out what the issues are with the current arrangements?
• Understand the user journey – work with homeless people already in receipt of services to carry out pathway mapping to understand their experiences, which services they interact with and what support would help them • Carry out an audit of case files from across different agencies to understand the issues being faced by the services and the factors behind decisions • Develop a multiple cause diagram to understand the factors involved in people becoming multiply excluded, and the links between them • Analyse complaints data from the police about crime levels • Use networks to identify best practice
What are the outcomes you want to achieve?
• For these individuals to have somewhere safe and warm to live and to have regular meals • For these individuals to access general healthcare and welfare benefits • For these individuals to get support in relation to dependency and mental health • To reduce the perceived and actual increased levels of crime within the local community • To reduce the number of emergency admissions of multiply excluded homeless people
How could you design an integrated intervention to deliver these outcomes?
• Use an AI approach to build on what the user mapping identified as good about current support • Use a creative thinking approach with staff and users to generate new ideas about a different way of supporting individuals • Develop a theory of change model to understand what the initiative would achieve and what the benefits would be

cont.

What might an integrated initiative look like?

A solution to the issue was to commission a local housing association to run a hostel that is able to cope with challenging behaviour. This will be achieved through:
- higher than usual staffing levels
- staff having additional training
- a specialist health team undertaking clinics in the hostel
- joint working with crisis mental health teams
- a multi-disciplinary team formed round each individual with a named care coordinator
- a multi-agency steering group with representatives from each key agency

Which services would need to be involved?

- Homeless services
- Community mental health team
- Community addictions service
- Local authority social work team
- Probation Service
- Police

Increasing numbers of older people are being admitted to A&E

There are concerns regarding the increased use of the acute hospital by older people with multiple morbidities, including those with dementia. This is leading to higher attendances at A&E and rates of readmission. There is also a need to reduce admissions of older people to residential and nursing home care from hospital whilst ensuring that there are not increases in people waiting for discharge.

How would you find out what the issues are with the current service?

- Use a Pareto diagram to understand the factors at play and the impact they have to identify where to focus resources
- Develop a cause and effect diagram to understand why increasing numbers of older people are presenting at A&E
- Undertake user pathway mapping to gain an understanding of the causes of entry and readmission

What are the outcomes you want to achieve?

- To enable people who experienced a short-term health or social crisis to return to their previous levels of independence
- To slow the rate of deterioration in the physical and mental health of people with long-term conditions
- To reduce the use of A&E and readmissions to hospital
- To reduce entry to long-term residential and nursing care
- To maintain (reduce) numbers of delayed discharges

How could you design an integrated intervention to deliver these outcomes?

- Gather best practice from existing approaches
- Use an experience-based design (EBD) approach to work with patients and their families to design a different approach
- Use de Bono's 'Six Thinking Hats' to generate creative ways of addressing the issues identified
- Use a 'safe-fail experiment' with one bed in a community hospital
- Create a theory of change model to design how a different approach would lead to improved outcomes

What might an integrated initiative look like?

A community-based rehabilitation and support service that seeks to enable people's timely discharge from hospital and to avoid readmission within 28 days, run by the acute hospital, and involving:
- community therapy services
- a reablement service with specialist home carers
- intermediary care beds in a community hospital
- social workers for hospital discharge (seconded into an acute trust)

Which services would need to be involved?

- Community therapy services
- District nursing
- Local authority social work team
- Reablement team
- Sheltered housing services
- Social care providers
- Preventative services delivered by the voluntary sector
- General practice
- Ambulance service
- Community leisure and education resources
- Out-of-hours health services

With strong links to a 'hospital to home' befriending service run by a local voluntary sector group, and access to a flat in a sheltered housing scheme that can be used for short stays prior to someone's own accommodation being available

There are high rates of type 2 diabetes in the South Asian community

The local area, which has a predominantly South Asian community, has high rates of type 2 diabetes. This is resulting in high rates of demand on secondary care diabetes services and other complications such as obesity and depression.

How would you find out what the issues are with the current service?

- Consult with older people from the South Asian community, using an advocacy group, to understand levels of awareness of the causes of type 2 diabetes
- Undertake user pathway mapping of a sample of 30 patients from the point of diagnosis
- Develop a cause and effect diagram based on the user pathway work
- Ask the neighbouring clinical commissioning group (CCG) with a similar population but lower rates of type 2 diabetes to conduct a three-day peer review of the service, in return for a reciprocal peer review in an area where they were performing better

What are the outcomes you want to achieve?

- To improve general awareness of the local community regarding the risk of diabetes through lifestyle and diet
- To target those at higher risk of developing diabetes with focused healthy living support
- To undertake diagnosis and if necessary insulin initiation in general practice rather than in the acute setting
- To encourage those with diabetes to self-manage their condition and avoid worsening and complications

cont.

How could you design an integrated intervention to deliver these outcomes?
• Commission local university to do a rapid evidence review into what works around diabetes prevention • Hold an Open Space session with people from across the public sector, third sector organisations and users and their families to identify issues and potential solutions • Use the de Bono 'Six Thinking Hats' approach within a multi-disciplinary team meeting • Develop a theory of change model to understand how the initiative would achieve the outcomes
What does the integrated initiative look like?
GP surgeries will offer an enhanced diabetic service that includes the following: • regular sessions from consultants and specialist nurses from the acute setting • consultants will jointly review patients with more complex diabetes with GPs with less confidence • monthly group case discussion with GPs and practice nurses who are more confident in which particular cases they bring for discussion • practice nurses will take on an additional health promotion role with support from dieticians • third sector organisation will provide sessions with a physical activity worker through a public health grant
Which services are involved?
• Federated general practices • Diabetic team in acute setting • Practice nurses • Community and religious groups • Local leisure and education services • Dietician service • Public Health department • Sheltered accommodation service for Asian elders • Voluntary and community support services for the local Asian community

Chapter 3

Engaging and Involving Individuals and Communities

Before we start thinking about why and how we should engage and involve patients, service users and carers, it is worth noting that there is some real ambiguity about the terms that people use to describe both those involved in these kinds of activities, and the activities themselves. For a start, it is difficult to agree a common term to describe someone receiving a health or social care service – are people patients, service users, clients, consumers or customers? In some cases, people who have had a disease, or condition, refer to themselves as survivors, so there are stroke survivors, cancer survivors and mental health survivors. Those looking after people in need of care are generally referred to as carers, but may also be referred to as care-givers.

When it comes to the activities we are going to talk about in this chapter, they are variously described as, amongst others, involvement, engagement, participation, collaboration, co-production and lay representation, or by the abbreviations PPI (public and patient involvement) and PPE (public and patient engagement). People are described as exercising their right to choice, voice and exit strategies in their interaction with health and social care, and we gather their experiences, we ask them for their evaluation of services, we empower them, and we measure their satisfaction. We also provide patient-centred care, person-centred care, individual care planning and negotiated care, and we expect people to self-care and to self-manage!

It can all become a bit of a minefield, but the important thing is to think carefully about what role someone is in at any point of time, what it is they are doing at any point in time, and to be consistent in your own use of terminology.

In this book we use the term 'service user' to refer to someone actively in receipt of a health or social care service, regardless of the nature of that service, and 'citizen' to refer to someone who is not actively in receipt of a service but in all likelihood has been at some point in time and may be again at some future point. We also use the term 'carer' to mean anyone either actively involved in the act of non-paid care-giving to an individual, or with responsibility for the welfare of an individual, such as a parent or guardian.

We use the term 'engagement' to refer to the process by which people are encouraged or facilitated to be interested in health and social care services, and their own health and wellbeing, and 'involvement' to mean their active participation in a specific activity.

We now come to the thorny issue of representativeness in engagement and involvement. There is a frequent argument used by some that an involvement activity isn't legitimate or credible because it isn't 'representative', or the participants themselves aren't representative. Concerns about representativeness are sometimes used to marginalise or discredit people's voices, especially when they are challenging the status quo. But what do they actually mean when people say something isn't representative?

They often mean that the people involved don't reflect the demographics either of the local community, or of service users in a statistical sense. For example, if you held an event that was specifically intended to gather the views of older people using day care services, of course you would want people there who were older who might use the service, but it might not be as important to have participants who statistically reflected the gender and ethnicity of the local older age community.

Whether those who are participating are representative of the group or community as a whole in a statistical sense is a contested concept – services might emphasise demographic correspondence, but service users themselves might emphasise the importance of empathy, shared experiences and local connections as being more important than statistical representativeness.

In any case, does statistical representativeness guarantee that the full range of views and experiences will be offered? For example, regarding older people's views on day care services, you might want to ensure that there are people there who have used the services for a while, people who have chosen not to, and people who have used them but who have stopped going, so you can understand the reasons for each scenario. You might also want to ensure that there are people there with and without disabilities, those living alone, and those living with others.

Is it also reasonable to expect a small number of individuals to fully represent all others? We know that service users often report feeling uncomfortable about this. Some argue that it is not representation of individuals that is important, but representation of the range of discursive positions within society, and therefore diversity and inclusion are better goals than representativeness per se.

Now we have covered some of the minefields in terminology, the rest of this chapter covers the following themes:

- Why do we engage and involve service users, carers and citizens?

- What activities do we engage and involve service users, carers and citizens in?

- What are the barriers to engaging and involving people in integrated initiatives?

- Which factors enable engagement and involvement?

- What are the key stages of involvement?

Why do we engage and involve service users, carers and citizens?

Engaging and involving service users, carers and citizens in health and social care have become key policy objectives internationally over the last few decades. This policy direction started with debates about empowerment for people with mental health problems and people with learning and physical disabilities in the 1980s and early 1990s, and continued through the 1990s, with debates about delivering health and social care services that would meet the needs of service users rather than meeting the needs of those who worked in them or ran them.

Over the intervening time, many policies have been introduced to encourage greater engagement and involvement of service users, carers and citizens in both health and social care services, and to encourage people to become fully engaged in their own health and wellbeing. Various organisations have been established to support active public involvement in health and social care. These policies and organisations facilitate the development of health and social care services where people have a far greater range of choices, and of information about services to enable those choices; and for a service that has better and more regular sources of information about people's preferences and opinions on the care and services they receive.

A whole range of reasons is given for engaging and involving people, and evidence supports many of these reasons, although the quality of that evidence is sometimes limited. In essence, however, there are two main reasons: the first is that engagement and involvement is 'an end in itself' – this refers to the rights-based argument and is concerned with people's self-determination and autonomy over their own health and wellbeing. This view of engagement and involvement challenges the traditional primacy of the professional by equalising power imbalances.

It is also suggested that involving citizens in decisions about which services are funded and how they are delivered means that such decisions will be better, fairer, more transparent and more democratically legitimate. This kind of involvement requires that citizens take some responsibility for decisions that affect society as a whole, particularly where there are difficult decisions to be made around ethical dilemmas, such as choices between funding services for one group of people over another. It is also suggested that there are educative benefits in this kind of involvement as it promotes more realistic public expectations about how much services cost and what can be afforded.

The second reason is that engagement and involvement is a 'means to an end' – this is based on the view that it leads to improved services that are more responsive to users' needs and are of a higher quality. This second reason is also recognised as leading to better outcomes for individuals, such as better compliance with medication or treatment regimes, and care decisions and treatment plans that are more appropriate and acceptable for the individual, through the sharing of knowledge and understanding amongst all parties. This kind of involvement can lead to improved psychological outcomes too, such as increased confidence in care recommendations, higher levels of satisfaction with the care received and better psychological adaption to illness or life circumstances.

The first reason is described as the 'democratic approach', where the focus is more about improving people's lives, by people having more say over the services they use and more control over their lives in general, whilst the second reason is often referred to as a 'consumerist approach', where the focus is the service system, the objective of which is to get service user, carer and citizen input to inform services and provision. It is, of course, possible that engagement and involvement activities may satisfy the needs of both democratic and consumerist approaches concurrently. However, for convenience, this chapter focuses on the second of these models, the consumerist approach, and Chapter 6 subsequently considers the first model, the democratic approach.

It is important to understand whereabouts on the spectrum between these approaches you are pitching your engagement or involvement activity, as this will determine whom you engage with and how you go about involvement. It is also important at the outset to match people's expectations to whereabouts on the spectrum their input is going. Whichever approach you are tending towards, though, it is important to remember that the activity must be meaningful for people and should make a difference, either to the individual or to the experience of receiving a service.

What activities do we engage and involve service users, carers and citizens in?

It is helpful to think about these kinds of activities occurring at different levels – for example, are we asking people to be involved in activities that will affect them as individuals, or are we asking people to be involved in providing their views on national policies and developments? Building on the micro, meso and macro framework introduced in Chapter 1, involvement can be thought of as occurring at the following levels:

- *Micro* – the involvement of the individual service user for their own benefit.

- *Meso* – the involvement of a group of service users for the benefit of a service.

- *Macro* – the involvement of the community, or citizens more widely, at a strategic level, whether across a whole system or at a national level.

It should also be recognised that an involvement continuum exists across these levels, but for the sake of simplicity, Table 3.1 shows what kinds of activities might occur at each level.

Although all organisations will be doing some form of engagement or involvement activity, many will not be doing this systematically, and probably most organisations would say they found engagement and involvement activities challenging.

Common concerns include how much it will cost to do properly, how to select people to take part, what methodologies or approaches to use, how to use the data that is gathered from these activities, and how to demonstrate that the activity has had any impact on the organisation, or for the individuals involved. These are all legitimate concerns and need careful thought, but before an organisation begins to involve service users, carers or citizens, it needs to take a step back from the overwhelming urge to 'do something' and think about the purpose of involving people. It is only in identifying the purpose of engagement and involvement that organisations can answer all the other questions above.

Table 3.1: Engagement and involvement activities at different levels

Micro	Meso	Macro
Self-management	Governance of services	Establishing values and ethical principles
Evaluation, e.g. feedback	Quality assurance of services	
Safety, e.g. prompting hand-washing, or raising awareness of allergies	Developing policy	Developing policy
Research	Consultation on plans for major service change	Consultation on plans for major service change
Shared decision-making and care planning	Allocating resources locally	Allocating resources strategically
Exercising choice – of provider, location, etc.		
Co-production	Co-production	

What are the barriers to engaging and involving people in integrated initiatives?

We cannot talk about engagement and involvement without introducing the concept of power, as this helps explain the nature of the relationship between individuals and the state and statutory organisations more widely, but also between individuals and health and social care professionals or systems. It also helps us think about why things don't always work as we had hoped they would.

Power theories help us to understand who is 'allowed' or not 'allowed' to be engaged or involved, and what the parameters of that activity are. For example, are people able to make their own decisions, or has a decision about something already been made and people are just being asked to support it? Are people offered a choice but only from a limited range of options pre-determined by someone else? Do people even believe they have a legitimate right to be asked for their view or opinion about something in the first place?

These different manifestations of power are likely to be apparent in all involvement or engagement activities and at all stages, from the initial idea that perhaps people ought to have a say in what is happening to the means by which the outcomes of the activity are publicised and promoted. One of the most obvious ways in which an organisation or individual professional can exercise power is to claim that people are not interested in being involved in decisions that may affect their lives. It is therefore appropriate to consider why this attitude prevails.

Do people want to be engaged and involved?

When asked about their motivations, people often say that they have become involved in providing feedback, or attending meetings, because they want to make a difference, or that they want to change things for the better or to give something back to a service that has helped them or those close to them. However, in spite of this altruistic desire from many people to be involved, surveys and other research suggest that actual involvement is lower than the amount of involvement people say they would like. There are a number of reasons why this might be the case.

The first, and most important reason is that people think their involvement will not make any difference to what happens. It's the 'Why bother? They won't take any account of what I've got to say and they'll do what they want to do anyway!' response, which we've probably all heard said to us, and probably all said ourselves at some point about giving feedback or our opinions on something. This perceived lack of influence relates directly to the power theories discussed previously – if people think they have no power to change anything, why would they bother to spend their time and effort getting involved?

The second important point to come out of these surveys and research is that people want decisions about the provision of health and social care services to be more open and accountable, but when it comes to complex decisions, people are more willing to give responsibility to professionals to make these decisions. This might be particularly the case where there may be trade-offs to make between the benefits of centralising some very specialised services to ensure expertise in these services, but the disbenefits of people not having a local service. And even when people feel they are not best placed to make the final decision, they still want their opinion to be taken into account.

The third point to note is that people often need practical support to be engaged and involved. This might mean that people need more information to help them make decisions, but it also means that they might need someone to take them to meetings, or they might want to attend events at different times to suit their personal circumstances. Practical support may mean that people have their travel expenses paid or costs of a child minder, or carer, covered whilst they are taking part in some activity.

'Professionalisation' of participants

The 'professionalisation' of participants is another issue that crops up again and again when talking about involvement. At the heart of both this and the concern over representativeness lies the issue of the 'typicality' or 'ordinariness' of those taking part. You will have probably heard the phrase 'the usual suspects', which means that the same people keep coming along to involvement activities. It is often used quite pejoratively in a way that suggests these individuals have some kind of involvement compulsion or are 'hangers-on'. At the same time, participants in involvement activities might be criticised for lacking particular knowledge or understanding of a clinical or technical issue. There is therefore a real tension between asking someone to take part in something because they have a level of expertise on a particular subject, that is, they have been caring for someone with a mental illness for years, or because you want the view of 'Joe/Jo Public'. Are you therefore looking for 'experience-based experts' or publically legitimate representatives?

It is also worth raising here whether it is actually feasible for someone to be completely objective or impartial about an issue, because we all have a particular view on life as a result of our personality, our experiences and the influence of people around us. This idea of complete impartiality is a contested subject and underlies debates about the partisan nature of participants in involvement activities. However thoughtfully you go about involvement, there remains the likelihood that you will leave out someone or some group.

Other barriers to effective involvement

Apart from those issues mentioned, a range of other issues might prevent people from wanting to take part in an engagement or involvement activity, or might make it more difficult for the activity to be meaningful to people, or for it ultimately to have some sort of impact and to make a difference.

These can include the real or imagined existence of a paternalistic culture in health and social care services, which might either actively discourage involvement, or might affect people's underlying assumptions about what will happen if they 'make a fuss' about something they are not happy with or that hasn't gone right for them.

Trust is an important aspect of engaging and involving people, and both sides have to learn to develop trust in each other to make the relationship work well. It is all too easy for service users, carers and citizens to lose trust in an individual or an organisation when things go wrong. It's often the little things that frustrate and annoy, and when taken together can lead people to disengage. For example, if someone arrives for a meeting and no one is expecting them because someone has forgotten to put their name down on a list, it creates an immediate barrier. If a service user needs wheelchair access to attend an event but this hasn't been picked up, it creates another barrier.

There may also be some very unrealistic expectations from both sides about what an engagement or involvement activity is likely to achieve. An organisation might think that it is reasonable to ask people to give their opinions about complex service changes without providing them with the right kind of preparation, or people might think they are able to design a new building when all they are being asked to comment on is the colour of the walls. If expectations aren't dealt with at the outset, it is likely to lead to frustration from both sides, which ultimately will affect how the next activity is viewed and whether people will want to take part.

If the environment is financially challenging, then individuals and organisations will need to make decisions about what activities they prioritise. It is likely that the delivery of services will be prioritised above other activities, and that activities such as engagement and involvement will be seen as 'nice to do', rather than 'need to do'. There is an assumption that these kinds of activities cost a lot of money, and, of course, some activities can take a lot of time and resources, but other activities need not break the bank if they are well thought out and well planned and are systematised. For example, it is worth investing in some software and training to design online questionnaires as this might be used many times over, and other organisations such as charities might sponsor events if they are able to have a stand and some promotional literature available on the day. Difficult operating environments should lead to creative solutions, rather than being a reason to stop doing things.

You may also have to be creative in how you work with people in different ways. It is quite likely that at times service users may not be well enough to take part in activities, or may not feel 'up to it' for whatever reason. Recognising that this is a consequence of the environment, and not the individual, and being flexible enough to adapt your plans, is important. As well as people's health and wellbeing affecting their ability to engage and get involved, people's level of health literacy can be seen as a barrier to accessing activities. In simple terms, you might need to think about how to provide people with materials in a range of languages, easy-to-read versions or braille, or you might need a signer to help at events or meetings. But you will also need to take into account the specifics of health and social care language – will you be using terminology that people will understand, will you be using jargon or acronyms that are obvious to you but not a lay person, or will you be talking about concepts that are difficult for most people to grasp, such as their risk of developing a particular disease or condition, or what randomisation in a clinical trial means?

Which factors enable engagement and involvement?

We've talked a lot about the barriers to engaging and involving people, so now it's time to think about what facilitates engagement and involvement. The CLEAR framework (Lowndes, Pratchett and Stoker 2006) is a really helpful and simple way of thinking this through (see Table 3.2), and sets out what is required from organisations and individuals for each factor.

Table 3.2: The CLEAR framework

Can do	Have the resources and knowledge to participate	Capacity building, training and support
Like to	Have a sense of attachment that reinforces participation	Building visibility, trust, relationships
Enabled to	Be provided with the opportunity for participation	Investing in infrastructure, groups and networks
Asked to	Mobilise by official bodies or voluntary groups	Opportunities that are appealing, engaging and appropriate; getting the 'ask' right
Responded to	See evidence that their views have been considered	Feedback on how decisions were made and views were considered

We have already talked a little bit about the 'Can do' by providing people with the practical support to be involved, whether this involves providing information or addressing logistical challenges. As regards the 'Like to', we mentioned earlier that people become involved with activities for a number of reasons, but building relationships and trust is crucial. Seeing involvement as a 'one-off' activity and only asking people to participate in something when you have a problem to solve, or a regulatory requirement to meet, will probably make some people feel rather used, so try to ensure that your involvement activity is something regular, continuous and systematised. Following on from this, involvement should be something that people enjoy doing and see a value in. The 'Asked to' suggests that people need to be 'mobilised' and to see a purpose in what they are being asked to do – this goes back to the point about involvement activities being meaningful. We consider the 'Enabled to' and 'Responded to' in more detail in the next section that looks at different stages in the process of involvement.

What are the key stages of involvement?

Stage 1: Determining the purpose of involvement

Before you jump in and start organising a workshop event, or start designing a questionnaire, be really clear about why you are doing this. You might intuitively think it's a good idea to do some involvement work (and it is!), but if you're not clear about the purpose, you won't know what the best approach is, who to involve and how, what to tell people about why you are asking them to do something for you, and what you will do with the answers you get or the data you gather (see Case example 3.1).

Asking yourself a series of questions as follows should help:

- Who will be using the information you collect? Will you be sharing the information with policy-makers and professionals, or service users, carers or citizens?

- At what level are you looking for involvement? Are you looking to involve people at the micro, meso or macro level? Do you want to know about strategic or operational issues?

- Whose issues are you asking for information on? Are you asking people to give you information to meet your agenda, or are you asking people what their agenda is?

- How will information be analysed? Do you have the analytical skills to analyse complicated quantitative data from surveys, or have you got software to help you? Do you have the time to analyse lots of qualitative information, and how will you draw together and analyse information from lots of different sources such as post-it notes, flip charts or drawings from a workshop event, for example?

- Will the information be summarised or aggregated? Depending on the answer to this, will the information still be meaningful to everyone you will share it with if it is summarised?

- How will decisions subsequently be made? Do you know what the process is by which the information you gather will affect decision-making?

- Is the involvement instrumental or symbolic? (The above questions and prompts generally assume that the involvement activity is instrumental and designed to meet a specific purpose. However, there may be a symbolic element to involvement, and that this is a means by which people's views are seen to be valued, or there may be some therapeutic value attached – 'tell us what has happened to you and it will get it off your chest'. If the purpose of involvement is either of the above, proceed with extreme caution. Symbolic gestures may make the organisation feel good, but if there is no tangible outcome for participants, it could do more harm than good in terms of your long-term relationship with service users, carers and citizens.)

Case example 3.1: Commissioning support services in Edinburgh

The City of Edinburgh Council, NHS Lothian, carer organisations and carers came together through a working group to redefine their strategic approach to commissioning support services for carers. The development of a three-year joint carers strategy for 2014–17 involved a consultation with carers on their priorities and the support they required. The approach set outcomes for carers at the centre of the new strategy.

To produce the strategy, the working group used the Wisconsin Logic Model[1] as a planning and evaluation tool. This approach brings detail to broad goals, helps identify gaps in strategies, is outcomes-focused, and makes underlying assumptions explicit. In order to ensure that all members of the working group knew how to work with the model, specific training was given to bring everyone up to the same level of

---

1   See www.uwex.edu/ces/pdande/evaluation/pdf/lmcourseall.pdf

knowledge and understanding about its application. The working group discussions were also independently facilitated.

Once six priority themes were agreed, the working group identified a set of questions under each theme on which it sought feedback from carers, including suggestions as to what type of support was needed under each heading. Written and online questionnaires were developed, and a number of consultations were held. The feedback from these events was fed directly back into the development of the strategy.

What does this case example tell us?

» The purpose of the involvement activity was clear to all those involved – it was to develop a new carers strategy, focused on carers' own priorities.

» The use of any specific tool or mechanism within involvement activities must be carefully thought through, with the development needs of all those involved in the activity appropriately addressed.

» Even though the working group involved carer organisations and carers, it recognised the benefits of consulting more widely to allow for a broader range of perspectives to be considered and for the emerging priorities to be confirmed.

Stage 2: Determining who is the focus of involvement

Again, it might be useful to ask yourself a series of questions, to be clear who is the focus of involvement – individuals or groups. There is also the scenario whereby people may offer their opinions and ideas informally, i.e. outside of any formal kind of involvement activity such as a survey exercise or a consultation event. A service user might provide you with feedback whilst you are visiting them at home to undertake an assessment, or as part of another professional contact. You will need to think about how you capture this information and ultimately how it is used. Otherwise, think about the following points:

• Do you want to target specific groups of people as 'experts by experience', or do you want participants who represent a broader range of experiences and perspectives?

• Is statistical representativeness an issue?

- Who are the seldom-heard groups or individuals in the area you are exploring?

- Is it going to be important for respondees/participants to be anonymous, and do you need to maintain confidentiality about their involvement?

- Will participants have the competence and capacity to take part? (Put simply, 'competency' refers to the mental ability and cognitive capabilities required to execute a specific task rationally, whereas 'capacity' refers to an individual's psychological abilities – specifically, their ability to understand, appreciate and manipulate information and to form rational decisions.)

- How can you ensure you are accessing participants who are likely to be supportive and challenging? (Be sure to not just seek the inclusion of people who are likely to tell you what you want to hear.)

It is also important in many instances to understand the views and experiences of people who do not access or use services. If you involve people who are not service users but who are eligible to be, and have chosen specifically not to do so, you will get very different views from those who do use the service in question. It is, of course, more difficult to identify who these people are, and will require a more creative approach to engagement. It is quite possible that people choose not to access or use a service because they do not have a sense of attachment to the organisation providing the service, or may actively choose not to identify as a service user – this means you will have to work first to establish trust.

Stage 3: Which engagement or involvement approach to use

So, let's imagine that you are clear about the purpose of your involvement activity and you know who you wish to involve. You now need to turn your attention to the approach and methodology. Table 3.3 provides a simple example of three approaches to engagement and involvement – the provision of information, consultation and participation – and examples of different methods you could use, such as information leaflets, surveys and citizens' juries.

Table 3.3: Three approaches to engagement and involvement

	Information	Consultation	Participation
Flow of information	One-way	One-way	Two-way
Purpose?	Letting people know and raising awareness about a change to an existing service	Getting a snapshot of people's views on proposals for a change to an existing service	Engaging in dialogue or negotiation to change national policies on paying for services
Who?	Service users of the specific service	Members of the local community	Citizens
How?	Leaflets, websites, local media, roadshows, noticeboards, newsletters	Surveys, focus groups, public meetings	Opinion polls, discussion forums on social media, petitions

There is, of course, a whole range of methods by which you could engage and involve people, and there are advantages and disadvantages to them all. Table 3.4 sets out the main methods and their strengths and weaknesses to give you a sense of when it might be appropriate to use them. Generally speaking, of course, an organisation will be using a range of methods all the time, as there is no one method that is acceptable, or appropriate, to all people, in all circumstances, and at all times; a range of methods is required to maximise response rates, increase representation of a range of experiences and viewpoints, and to avoid bias. Think of it like a toolbox of methods, and choose the one(s) that you think fits best with the 'why', 'what' and 'who'.

It is also worth bearing in mind that people can sometimes feel overwhelmed by requests for information or involvement, and so it is important not to bombard service users, carers and citizens with multiple requests. This is especially important when you are working in an integrated care setting, and a number of organisations might want to lead these kinds of activities. It is important therefore that you are clear which organisation, team or department has responsibility for these kinds of activities, so that energy and costs are not duplicated, and goodwill is not jeopardised.

Table 3.4: Main methods of engagement and involvement, and their strengths and weaknesses

	Approach (e.g. information, consultation, participation)	Volume reach	Provision of quantitative data	Provision of qualitative data	Speed of response	Real-time information	Low-cost	User-friendly	Reporting of sensitive information
Roadshows	Information	✓	✓	✓				✓	
Leaflets	Information	✓	✓	✓				✓	
Newsletters	Information	✓	✓	✓				✓	
Public meetings	Information Consultation		✓	✓	✓	✓			
Self-administered questionnaire/ survey (not online)	Consultation	✓	✓✓	✓			✓	✓	✓✓
Comment/feedback cards	Consultation	✓		✓	✓	✓	✓✓	✓✓	
Hand-held devices	Consultation	✓✓	✓✓		✓✓	✓	✓	✓	
Touch-screen kiosks	Consultation	✓	✓✓		✓✓	✓	✓	✓	
Online questionnaires	Consultation	✓✓	✓✓	✓	✓		✓✓	✓	✓✓
Telephone interviewing	Participation			✓	✓			✓	
Depth interview (service user story)	Participation			✓✓	✓			✓✓	✓
Peer researchers	Participation			✓✓				✓✓	✓
External websites (NHS Choices, Patient Opinion)	Consultation Participation	✓		✓	✓		✓	✓	
Focus group	Consultation Participation			✓✓				✓	
Online communities	Information Consultation Participation	✓		✓	✓		✓	✓	
Social media – Facebook	Information Consultation Participation	✓		✓	✓		✓	✓	✓
Social media – Tweets	Information Consultation Participation	✓	✓	✓	✓✓	✓	✓	✓	
Citizens' juries	Information Consultation Participation			✓					
Experience-based design/co-production	Information Consultation Participation			✓				✓	

Whatever method(s) you choose to use, good practice dictates that you test it out first. This means that if you ask people to complete a survey, 'pilot' the questions first – do your pilot respondents understand what information they are being asked for, and will they interpret things in the same way as the person who has designed the questionnaire? The same will be true if you are using a topic guide in an interview. It is also worth thinking about the increasing use of technology as a proxy for human contact – what you might gain from convenience and speeding up the process, you might lose in engagement and developing rapport with some groups of people.

There are also advantages and disadvantages in collecting information from people at the point at which they are receiving a service – 'real time' – and collecting information some time after they have received a service – 'retrospective'. It has been suggested that collecting information in 'real time' gives the organisation and its staff more motivation to act, because the information is fresh and it is easier to determine cause and effect. It is therefore easier to prevent issues from becoming problems and to improve the overall experience for others. There are, however, disadvantages in seeking 'real-time' feedback, partly because reflection is an important element of giving feedback on an experience, but also because there is a phenomenon called the 'positivity of response bias', which means that some people may provide more positive feedback during an episode of care because there are inherent difficulties in talking about poor experiences and a concern that negative feedback will affect ongoing care, as they will be viewed as troublemakers, or as difficult people to deal with. Also, however, some people have a deep-rooted psychological need to remain optimistic, and do not want to contemplate that things might not be going as well as they could.

Roadshows, leaflets and newsletters need to be engaging – remember that involvement, in whatever guise, should be a pleasurable experience for people. This also means that events should not be intimidating or overwhelming, thus preventing people from wanting to contribute. Public meetings, and in particular, formal public meetings, can be very bound by procedures and rules, making them very user-unfriendly. But if this is the means by which you are required to involve people on occasions, try to think about how the meetings can be made to feel more inclusive – perhaps by arranging the seating in a semi-circle, away from desks or tables, or by ensuring that the chair of the meeting is very skilled at making everyone's voices heard.

When it comes to methods such as postal questionnaires or surveys, response rates can be variable according to demographics, though in general, response rates to postal surveys are declining. Anonymous questionnaires can lead to the disclosure of more sensitive information than you might otherwise receive, but the fact that they are anonymous means that people cannot be followed up for additional involvement, where this might seem appropriate.

Methods such as comment or feedback cards can provide extreme views, so that you are only told if someone has had a very good or very bad experience. A survey using electronic means such as hand-held tablets, or touch-screen kiosks, can provide a more nuanced set of responses, but the number of questions generated is nonetheless quite limited in number. However, the results from these kinds of devices are analysed automatically, which can save time, and negates the need for a specific set of analytical skills.

Online questionnaires or involvement activities involving social media can be used creatively, and the nature of online engagement often means a reduction in self-moderation and the disclosure of more sensitive information, which might be beneficial. People can also dip into and out of activities, as convenient. In addition, an interactive website can enable organisations to engage in a more participatory way with people, though this sort of dynamic interaction would require more management of the activity. And a further word of caution – in spite of the growth in home internet access, any online method will still disadvantage certain demographics such as older people and the socially disadvantaged, in terms of access, so think carefully about these methods.

Deliberation events are based on egalitarian principles, but it is important to be realistic that participants themselves may not always follow these principles in practice. Small group discussions tend towards the majority view, and power and professional and hierarchical status can influence the underlying assumptions of the group. An example of this kind of involvement activity is illustrated in Case example 3.2. The same can be true of focus groups, so it is important to consider sampling of participants carefully.

Face-to-face interviews and their subsequent analysis are the most inclusive method of involvement, but they are time-consuming to undertake and require skill to do well. The presence of the interviewer can also have a moderating effect on responses, so that participants may not always feel able to be as candid about their experiences, or their opinions, as they might be through other means. However, it is clear that people appreciate the human dynamic of this kind of interaction. These same kinds of issues are also relevant for telephone interviews, although powerful visual clues to what someone is really thinking or feeling will often be lost.

Case example 3.2: Review of Jersey's mental health services

When the State of Jersey's Department of Health and Social Services (DHSS) began its review of mental health services on the island in 2014, it made a conscious decision to involve citizens at the outset in its review, rather than wait until decisions had been made before consulting them. The methodology used was a citizens' panel that was managed and facilitated by external and independent experts. Vouchers were offered as incentives to people to take part, and the costs of childcare, travel, etc. were reimbursed.

It was essential to the success of the project that a diverse group of people was recruited to take part. This involved the distribution of 1000 letters inviting people to take part, randomly generated by the island's postal service. Invitations were also distributed through local organisations such as Mind Jersey and the Jersey Alzheimer's Association. Seventy people expressed an interest in taking part, from which 25 participants were purposively sampled to ensure variation by gender, ethnicity, age, geographical location and experience of using Jersey's mental health services. Thus the final sample included people who described themselves as using the services currently, those who had in the past, and those who had never used the island's mental health services.

The panel convened on four occasions across two weeks, meeting for two-and-a-half hours on a weekday evening. The first two sessions enabled people to think about the current system of support and what was working well and what was not working so well, and to share their life experiences. The third session drew on the expertise of mental health professionals to explore the evidence about what was known to work well in the delivery of mental health services elsewhere. The fourth session allowed participants to develop the building blocks they agreed were important for the development of a new strategy for the delivery of mental health services in Jersey.

What does this case example tell us?

» Members of the public were involved from the outset in the review, which demonstrates a commitment from the DHSS to equalise the power dynamics between the state and citizens.

» Although people were invited at random to take part, people self-selected in volunteering to take part. It is possible that this approach means that the voices of the most disadvantaged and least able to take part because of the level of support required to participate were not heard. However, including the charitable organisations and other local groups in the recruitment potentially went some way to mitigate for this.

» The scheduling of the sessions and the financial support offered were helpful in enabling people to participate.

» The activities at each session allowed people to contribute equally and meaningfully.

But whatever method you use, such as collecting information and data from people, or involving them in a citizens' jury (or panel) or co-production exercise, the act of involvement is only as good as the resulting action, which leads us nicely into the next section – how the organisation responds to the outputs from involvement.

Stage 4: How to respond to involvement outputs

Responding appropriately to involvement activities requires a willingness to be open and transparent and to be committed to the principles of involvement – for example, individuals and organisations will need to be able to respond objectively so that credence isn't only given to what the organisation might want to hear, but to everything that is being said.

Responding appropriately often also requires some specific insights and skills. The organisation may require some technical expertise to analyse data or information gathered to help interpret the outputs of the activity, and therefore translate these into outcomes. It is important to think at the outset whether the outputs of your activity are likely to be actionable. So, does your organisation have the capacity and capability to design, collate, analyse, interpret and act on engagement and involvement activities? We have already seen that the enthusiasm of people to be involved is related to their ability to change or to improve things for others. To maintain that sense of engagement, it is crucial to have some means by which you can tell people what difference their involvement has made (see Case example 3.3).

Case example 3.3: National Voices and the development of 'I' statements

The development of a narrative around what integrated care is from a user perspective is a good example of how participants were able to see the difference their input was making. In 2012, the NHS commissioned National Voices to work with it to co-produce a new definition of integration, taking the user perspective as the organising principle.

In order to do this, National Voices first reviewed its own set of 'I' statements that had previously been developed based on evidence and feedback from members of the organisation. These statements illustrated what good care might look like from the service user's perspective, that is, 'I don't want to have to repeat my story every time I see a different carer.' A workshop was then organised to test these statements out with health and social care professionals, policy-makers and individual service users and representatives from service user organisations. A second version of the statements was drafted and circulated to attendees. After further revision these were made public and additional feedback was sought. A second workshop in March 2013 reviewed all the feedback and agreed a third and final version in May 2013. Key revisions emphasised the service users' need for autonomy.

This narrative has become the source of measurement for people's experiences of coordinated care and is being used by NHS England to develop new questions for national surveys. It is also being used to develop measures for success for local commissioners.

What does this case example tell us?

» The involvement process allowed for iterative versions of the narrative to be developed based on participant feedback. This was a clear and transparent process.

» The exercise has had a visible impact nationally, and has been publicised by organisations such as The King's Fund.

Stage 5: Reviewing and improving the impact of involvement

It is a sad fact that we know very little about the achievements of involvement. The evidence base for demonstrating impact from engagement and involvement activities is limited and of poor quality in the main. Few studies define what they mean by involvement, and there is an absence of robust measurement of impact. In reality, there is a lack of valid, reliable instruments to measure impact and persistent issues with attribution, so that it is not always possible to isolate the effects of an involvement activity with the effects of another policy initiative. The literature is also weak in reporting the cost-effectiveness of engagement and involvement activity. Unfortunately, it becomes a vicious circle, for the fewer studies that describe the benefits of engagement and involvement on the delivery of services, the less likely organisations may be to give service users, carers and citizens a bigger voice in these matters.

There are a number of ways in which you can measure the impact of your own activities. These might include surveys, interviews or focus groups. They might also include documentary analysis – this could be of board or other meeting minutes to see how the outputs of involvement activities play into these decision-making fora, or observation of meetings to capture opinions about the difference engagement and involvement has made. Of course, impact can be felt in the short and longer term, or across different time points, and you will therefore need to use methods that recognise this. To add to the complexity, the impact of activities could be felt by participants, the organisation or third parties, the identity of whom might not be known either in the short term, or at all. This would be the case, for example, if an experience-based design (EBD) event led to improvements to services that would be felt by future service users.

So, what kinds of impact are we looking for from engagement and involvement activities? The list below is not exhaustive, but is designed to give you a sense of what you might be looking out for:

- development of trust between organisations and the people they serve

- changes to organisational culture and professional attitudes to service users and carers – this might include fostering better dialogue between parties and better shared decision-making opportunities

- services that better reflect the needs of patients, service users and carers

- changes to how people think, feel and behave in relation to their own health and wellbeing and the use of services

- development of new skills and confidence for patients, service users and carers

- development of new skills and confidence amongst staff.

Whatever impact you are hoping to achieve and whatever measures you use to assess whether it has been achieved, someone has to take responsibility for this final aspect of engagement and involvement on behalf of the organisation.

Chapter 4

Leading Self and Others

Leading a change programme is a challenging task. Developing person-centred, coordinated care in the face of long-standing fragmentation takes strong leadership that can build a consensus that there is a better way to operate, and be able to move resources where they are needed most, irrespective of traditional boundaries or ways of working. Holding this consensus together through the often-challenging practical steps to implementation is a big leadership challenge.

You may not be leading the entirety of the integration approach, but your role in developing a new approach for specific services requires the same level of understanding about effective leadership as those at the top of the organisations involved. This chapter therefore focuses on how to lead the change you need to implement *from where you are*. You may be working for a senior leader or project sponsor, with some decisions already made for you, but you will need to show leadership for the staff in your teams and those who need to deliver the change. Whilst Chapter 5 focuses on the process of change, this chapter focuses on the skills and personal approaches required to implement and sustain a successful change programme, and covers the following:

- How can you lead change when you're not in charge?

- What is the environment in which you are leading and the task to be done?

- What are the frameworks to help the leading of change in a complex environment?

- How can you develop resilience for self, and for your team?

How can you lead change when you're not in charge?

The concept of distributed or collaborative leadership has gained a lot of traction within the NHS and local government in recent years. With recognition of the complexity of the issues and the systems, there is a shift away from the concept of a hero leader at the top of an organisation who has all the answers. Arguably the kinds of challenges facing public services – which require work across boundaries and in the absence of formal authority – require more use of distributed leadership and less use of hierarchy. The implication of this approach is that senior leaders may expect those in middle management positions to act as leaders, and feel that they have given them the mandate to do so.

Characteristics of distributed leadership include:

- an emergent group or network of interacting individuals

- drawing on a variety of expertise distributed across the many, not the few

- leadership exercised not just by those with positional authority

- leadership exercised by anyone at any position in the hierarchy who takes responsibility for change.

Despite these aspirations for distributed leadership, managers still often feel caught in the middle – between the expectations of senior leaders at the top of the organisation and managing those who have to change and deliver services in a different way. Working in a middle management role, you may not feel that you are able to (or required to) exercise leadership. Yet these roles are often where a change programme succeeds or fails. Middle managers are the ones who not only have to buy into and deliver the vision set by senior leaders, but also need to share a compelling vision with their own teams, and ensure that the services deliver whilst in the middle of change, and that the details of how the change will happen are implemented. You may find yourself needing to influence and negotiate up the organisation, and with others inside and outside of your own organisation – people to whom you have no line management relationship. How can you exercise power without that position of power? It's useful to recognise that even if you are not in a formal position of power within an organisation, you may have alternative sources of power and influence (see Table 4.1).

Table 4.1: Different sources of power and influence

Types of power	Sources of power
Legitimate power (sometimes called 'authority' or 'formal' power)	All managers have some level of legitimate power – certain powers given to them in order to do their job effectively
Reward power	Managers have control over certain rewards, such as pay increases, promotions, work schedules, status symbols and recognition awards, which they can use to reward desirable behaviour
Coercive power	The opposite of reward power, based on the ability of the individual to sanction or prevent someone from obtaining desirable rewards
Expert power	From having knowledge that is valued by the organisation or individuals with whom the person interacts, e.g. expertise in a particular field or at problem-solving or performing critical tasks
Referent power	An individual who gains admiration, loyalty and emulation to the extent that they are able to influence others, e.g. having a vision, strong convictions about the correctness of the vision, confidence in their ability to deliver or realise the vision, or seen by their followers as agents of change
Connection or networking power	About who you know, vertically and horizontally, both within and outside the organisation, e.g. the 'Old Boys Club'. Networking power represents many of the political dynamics that make up organisations
Information power	A manager should have more information power than their team, but this may not be the case. An individual who is part of the 'grapevine' often has more accurate information than the manager

Source: Adapted from Hersey and Blanchard (1969)

So, as you can see from Table 4.1, you may have more power to effect change than you might think. Leading an integrated care initiative can complicate sources of power as these may not be transferable between the agencies involved (e.g. being a health specialist may not be seen as that important an 'expertise' to housing staff), or indeed, may add sources of power that were not previously available (e.g. being able to explain or agree to resources available through another agency). In undertaking this role, leaders of integrated care initiatives often need to be boundary spanners.

Boundary-spanning leadership can be defined as the capability to establish direction, alignment and commitment across boundaries in service of a higher vision or goal. As someone tasked with making integration real, it is likely that you will need to act as a boundary spanner between different professions and organisations. Potential roles and competencies of boundary spanners are described in Figure 4.1.

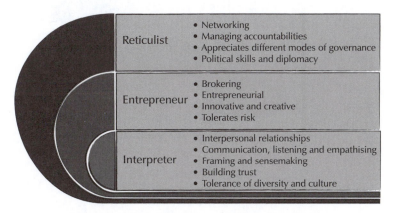

Figure 4.1: Roles and competencies of boundary spanners
Source: Based on Ernst and Chrobot-Mason (2010) and Ernst and Yip (2009)

These boundary-spanning roles may be key in integrating services, as they are able to cross the current organisational boundaries. Boundary-spanning roles such as reticulists are often not located at the top of the formal organisational hierarchy, but usually have good access to it. They are less bound by normal and accepted channels of organisational behaviour, and are encouraged or allowed to be unconventional. Their position and status within the hierarchy is such that they do not represent an explicit threat to top management, but are tolerated in the expectation that they can deliver solutions to complex problems. You may be able to recognise your role in acting as a boundary spanner, and be able to use that role to lead the change you are seeking to make.

To be a successful leader you not only need to understand leadership, but also the concept of followership. Usually when acting in a leadership role you are also acting as a follower, of the senior leaders who have set out the vision, or the programme manager for the overarching integration work, and you need to recognise that your teams are your followers. Grint and Holt (2011) suggest that where we are dealing with wicked issuesand complex adaptive systems, where there is a need to develop solutions together, instead of traditional compliant or technical followers who will carry out orders and processes, we need responsible followers who will take responsibility for their part in finding a solution to the issue (see Figure 4.2).

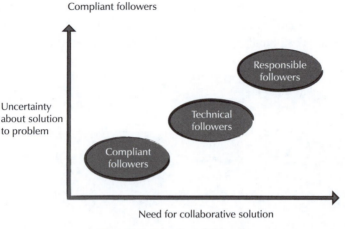

Figure 4.2: Compliant followership
Source: Adapted from Grint and Holt (2011)

But, as we often see in change programmes, followers may not always agree with the direction of travel, and may resist and contest the official line. Grint and Holt suggest a variety of outcomes here – people may deny the crisis and may rebel against the leadership (*mutineers*); some followers may deny the complex nature of their situation and continue to execute the procedures knowing they will not work ('work to rule' followers or *chronic followers*); and followers who deny the wicked nature of their situation and refuse to accept collective responsibility for it (*refuseniks*) (see Figure 4.3).

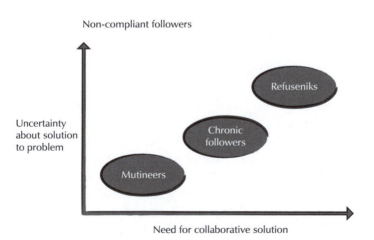

Figure 4.3: Non-compliant followership
Source: Adapted from Grint and Holt (2011)

A situation such as integrating services is likely to demand a high level of collective responsibility from followers. If you are in the situation of leading teams of different professionals, how can you work with them to create responsible followers who will work together to find the solutions? And what role are you playing in terms of being a follower of the overall vision?

What is the environment in which you are leading and the task to be done?

As discussed in Chapters 1 and 2, the aims of integrating health and social care are often manifold, dealing with people with complex lives and issues. Integration is often seen as a way of addressing 'wicked issues', which are those that are not caused by and cannot be solved by one part of the system. With wicked issues there is no easy, simple solution to the problem. The issues that you are trying to tackle through integrating your services are wicked issues (e.g. a young man with mental health problems who has no stable accommodation; a middle-aged Asian lady who has just been diagnosed with diabetes). Wicked issues are system problems and solutions, such as integrating services, and operate within a complex, adaptive system.

Tackling wicked issues means that there is often no simple, agreed answer. Stacey's (2009) model (see Figure 4.4) may offer a helpful framework that is relevant to the task of integrating health and social care. It suggests that there are different ways of leading or managing the implementation, depending on the levels of agreement over what to do, and high or low levels of certainty about what to do. Where we know what to do and there is agreement about it, we are in the 'box' of ordinary management, keeping the day job going. In most integration initiatives there will be some aspects where there is certainty and agreement about the way forward (e.g. which services will be integrated or maybe where a service might be co-located). This will require good management but is not a demanding leadership challenge. However, as we move into the realms of where we are not so sure what to do (e.g. how to develop an effective pathway or share data from across a range of organisations), the challenge is more uncertain and 'messy'. In terms of implementing integration, this means paying attention to the day job of good management, but also ensuring that you, and others, are comfortable within the ambiguity of the situation – encouraging experiments, remaining curious and not jumping to quick solutions, encouraging networking and conversations between teams, building new relationships, challenging held assumptions and containing the potentially high level of anxiety amongst staff. This may mean enabling action research types of approaches, creating small groups of multi-agency teams to work on specific aspects, and creating forums where people can create connections, and where those doing the work are able to develop and implement it.

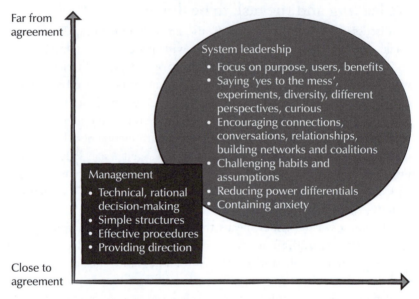

Figure 4.4: Certainty and agreement
Source: Adapted from Stacey (2009)

Heifetz *et al.* (2009) build on Stacey's work, and define two different types of problems: *technical* and *adaptive*. These require different leadership approaches. Expertise and good management can solve technical problems, whereas adaptive problems, such as poverty, inequality in health outcomes and drug abuse, require innovation and learning. Traditional management strategies are useful in dealing with technical problems, but in situations where beliefs and values come into play, such technical 'fixes' tend to exacerbate the problem. By definition, adaptive challenges involve a disparity between values and circumstances. The task of the leader is to close the gap. This may involve marshalling energy, resources and ingenuity to change the circumstances, but just as often it requires that people change their values. Leadership therefore consists 'not of answers or assured visions, but of taking action to clarify values' (Heifetz 1994). Good leaders know how to stimulate and contain the forces of invention and change, and to shift the process from one stage to the next. This is all very relevant for the task of integrating services, where you may need to help staff to change their values around issues such as, for example, levels of dependency.

Matland's (1995) model is a useful way of framing the type of policy implementation that you are involved in, based on the levels of conflict and ambiguity about the policy (see Tables 4.2 and 4.3). When implementing a complex change such as integration, there may be different contexts within one change programme. For example, there may be some policies in the low ambiguity/low conflict box, such as the creation of multi-disciplinary, neighbourhood teams where the end goal is clear and there is agreement about what the teams should consist of. These policies should be simple, administrative implementation. Other policies, such as the development of an integrated dementia pathway, may have high ambiguity because there will be different options, but low conflict as everyone agrees that it is the right thing to do. In these cases there is room to experiment about how the policy is implemented. Some major integration approaches, such as a structural merger, fall into the category of high conflict and low ambiguity – it is clear what is supposed to happen, but the level of conflict between the organisations is likely to lead to high conflict. Some policies, for example information sharing across organisations, fall into the category of high conflict and high ambiguity and are likely not to be implemented. In the realm of integration, it is likely that many of the changes fall into the context of the high ambiguity/low conflict approach, where there is usually general agreement from people within the system that integration is a good thing, but less clarity over exactly how to do it, and what the specific goals, processes, structures and technology to be used are, etc. There is often a focus on the what, rather than on the how.

Table 4.2: Conflict – ambiguity matrix

	Low conflict	High conflict
Low ambiguity	**Administrative implementation**	**Political implementation**
	Goals are given and the solution to the problem is known One organisation has the resources, capacity, information and capability to enact the policy There is a hierarchical process for implementation to follow Policy is clear at each level and there is agreement on policies and tasks Uniform outcomes across sites	Conflict over both goals and means Implementation process is a key area for conflict Outcomes are determined by distribution of power Compliance is not automatically forthcoming Monitoring of compliance is relatively easy
High ambiguity	**Experimental implementation**	**Symbolic implementation**
	Outcomes depend on which actors are involved and are hard to predict Variation in outcomes across different sites Opportunities for local agents to create local policies Compliance monitoring is low relevance Policy may become low priority	Salient symbols can produce high levels of conflict even when policy is vague Outcomes will depend on balance of local coalition strength Activities are difficult to monitor

Source: Adapted from Matland (1995)

Table 4.3: Conflict – ambiguity matrix relating to the diabetes scenario

	Low conflict	High conflict
Low ambiguity	**Administrative implementation**	**Political implementation**
	Creation of an enhanced diabetes service Regular sessions from consultants and specialist nurses from the acute hospital	Consultants will jointly review patients with more complex diabetes with GPs with less confidence Practice nurses to take on additional health promotion role with support from dieticians
High ambiguity	**Experimental implementation**	**Symbolic implementation**
	Involving community and religious groups and support services for the local Asian community in development and promotion of the service	Third sector organisation will provide physical activity worker sessions through a public health grant

Source: Adapted from Matland (1995)

What are the frameworks to help the leading of change in a complex environment?

When leading a complex change such as designing and implementing an integrated initiative, a different kind of leadership is needed from that of day-to-day service management. In this section we look at some of these different leadership approaches that you may want to use.

Transactional and/or transformational leadership

Kotter's (1990) work on transactional and transformational leadership is useful because it helps to distinguish the everyday management style of leadership from the transformational leadership that is often needed to make a large change programme happen. It may be that your role will require a combination of the two approaches and you move between the two as your implementation takes shape. You are likely to need to focus on the transactional tasks in order to build new teams and define and monitor budgets and outputs, but you will also need to pay attention to the transformative tasks of communicating the wider vision, motivating and inspiring new teams and giving people a sense of belonging within a newly formed team or organisation. You will need to ensure that you are giving sufficient attention to both aspects of leadership and keep the day job going whilst inspiring and motivating teams.

Table 4.4: Transactional and transformational leadership

	Transactional leadership	Transformational leadership
Creating an agenda	Planning and budgeting Developing a detailed plan of how to achieve results	Establishing direction: developing a vision that describes a future state and strategy of how to get there
Developing human resources (HR)	Organising and staffing: deciding which individual best fits each job and who can deliver the plan	Aligning people: getting people to understand and believe the vision
Execution	Controlling and problem-solving: monitoring results, identifying deviations from the plan and solving problems	Motivating and inspiring: satisfying people's needs for achievement, belonging, recognition, self-esteem and sense of control
Outcomes	Produces degree of predictability and order	Produces change

Source: Adapted from Kotter (1990)

Systems leadership

A systems leadership approach has recently gained traction, through work done by the Leadership Centre and The King's Fund on health services. Systems leadership can be defined as leadership across organisational and geopolitical *boundaries*, beyond individual professional *disciplines*, within a range of organisational and stakeholder *cultures*, and often without direct managerial *control*. The purpose of systems leadership is to *effect change for positive social benefit across multiple interacting and intersecting systems.*

Recent work carried out by the Advancing Quality Alliance (AQuA) with their Discovery Communities in the North West[1] identified the characteristics, skills and knowledge needed for systems leadership of integrated care, at every level (see Table 4.5).

Table 4.5: Skills and knowledge of systems leadership

Technical know-how	Service design
	Governance arrangements
	Innovative contracting and financial mechanisms
	Technologically 'savvy'
Improvement know-how	Systems thinking
	Improvement science
	Large-scale change
Personal effectiveness	Interpersonal skills and behaviours
	Coaching ability
	Visionary and participative style

AQuA then developed a programme of support for officers who were leading integrated initiatives to acquire the skills and knowledge set out above. Their reflection was that organisations themselves do not always offer appropriate support for staff trying to deliver radical change programmes, and so looking outside the organisation to what might be offered by partners or membership bodies may be beneficial. The learning from AQuA's work might be helpful in thinking through how to develop the leadership skills you need (see Case example 4.1).

---

1   Personal correspondence.

Case example 4.1: Advancing Quality Alliance's (AQuA) Discovery Community

AQuA's support programme for its Discovery Community put in place a blended approach that offered a variety of support. Initially a multi-agency team was brought together to explore where they were, where the differences were, different language, line management arrangements, accountability and risk. Together they undertook a baseline assessment of their readiness for change. Teams worked together over a period of several months to learn about improvement methods, to develop the technical skills to deliver change projects and build effective interpersonal relationships across diverse teams. AQuA found that time out together as a team was the most important ingredient, recognising that creating team spirit and trust takes time. It was clear that there needed to be an expectation that they wanted to create a team. The learning from the programme was that the process of the team coming together to discover, learn and plan collectively was as important as the technical and content knowledge that the teams acquired on the programme.

AQuA also offered team and individual coaching, and techniques to develop resilience.

What does this case example tell us?

»   Providing space to learn – creating a forum where ideas can be shared and tested, information is exchanged and in which leaders are not expected to know all the answers.

»   Focus on place – this can create a strong unifying element that can overcome some of the difficulties caused by differences within the system (e.g. language, professional training, accountability, appetite for risk).

»   Insatiable curiosity – the desire to understand (rather than know), to learn (rather than teach), to share (rather than compete) and to experiment (rather than stick to how things are always done).

Source: Weir and Fillingham (2014)

Goleman's leadership styles

We have looked at the dimensions of systems leadership, and within this there will be decisions to make about how best to lead at a particular point in the implementation process. Goleman's (2000) leadership styles suggest different approaches to 'getting things done', which can be chosen and utilised at the appropriate moment, just like choosing an appropriate golf club. Goleman also suggests the negative impacts that certain ways of leading may have on others (see Figure 4.5). So, for example, in taking forward integration, you may need a combination of authoritative and democratic approaches, to mobilise colleagues from across various organisations towards a vision, and to forge consensus through participation. You will need to bear in mind the impact of a leadership style on others, even if not your own approach; if the overriding approach from the organisation is one of pace-setting, this is likely to have a negative longer-term impact on the team, and on you, so you may want to offer an alternative leadership approach to alleviate the impact.

	Coaching	Pace-setting	Democratic	Affiliative	Authoritative	Coercive
Leader's approach	Develops people for the future	Sets high standards for performance	Creates consensus through participation	Creates harmony and builds emotional bonds	Mobilises people towards a vision	Demands immediate compliance
Most likely to say	'Try this'	'Do as I do, now'	'What do you think?'	'People come first'	'Come with me'	'Do what I tell you'
Emotional intelligence competencies	Develops others, empathy, self-awareness	Conscientious, drive to achieve, initiative, team leadership, communication	Collaboration, team leadership, communication	Empathy, builds relationships, communication	Self-confidence, empathy, change catalyst	Drive to achieve, initiative, self-control
When to use the approach	Help an employee improve performance or develop strengths	Get quick results from highly motivated and competent team	Build buy in and consensus or to get input from employees	Heal rifts in a team to motivate people in stressful circumstances	When changes require a new vision or clear direction is needed	In a crisis to kick start a turnaround, or with problem employees
Overall impact of approach	Positive	Negative	Positive	Positive	Most strongly positive	Negative

Figure 4.5: Leadership styles
Source: Adapted from Goleman (2000)

How can you develop resilience for self, and for your team?

In a complex world, where you need to understand the system, describe it to others, create a vision for the future and also deliver day-to-day services, you will need to ensure that you have the resilience to keep going, and to maintain your physical and mental wellbeing. In this section we discuss ways of developing and sustaining resilience, but we begin by thinking about how to identify when the pressure may be becoming too much to bear.

Recognising stress

A key technique to remaining effective and in control is to recognise when you are stressed. For those practitioners who have carried out the Myers-Briggs® type indicator (MBTI®) assessments, you may be familiar with the term 'being in the grip' (Quenk 1996). Many practitioners have carried out MBTI assessment and have an understanding of their personality 'type' (see Table 4.6). Each type has a pattern of behaviour that is displayed when the person is stressed. The key is to understand how this manifests itself, to share it with others so that they can also recognise it, and to understand the potential solutions there might be to address the issues. For those who know their type, we have set out the 'in the grip' behaviour and potential solutions below, in Table 4.6.

Table 4.6: 'In the grip' behaviour

Personality type	'In the grip' behaviour	Solution
ESTJ/ ENTJ	Hypersensitive to inner state, outbursts of emotion, fear of feeling	Allow time in the day to really feel emotions, talk to a good friend who will just listen and not offer advice
ISFP/ INFP	Judgements of incompetence, aggressive criticism, precipitous action	Allow behaviour to expire on its own, get feelings validated without someone trying to reason with them
ISTP/ INTP	Logic emphasised to an extreme, hypersensitive to relationships and feelings of rejection or disapproval, emotionalism	Others should respect their physical and psychological space, lighten responsibilities, and avoid asking them how they feel
ESFJ/ ENFJ	Excessive criticism, convoluted logic, compulsive search for truth	Solitude and journaling, new projects, others need to leave them alone
ESTP/ ESFP	Internal confusion, inappropriate attribution of meaning, grandiose vision	Make contingency plans, reassurance from others regarding 'dire' consequences, get help in setting priorities
INTJ/ INFJ	Obsessive focus on external data, over-indulgence in sensual pleasure, adversarial attitude towards the world	Time alone to recharge, reducing schedule, others should avoid offering advice or suggestions
ISTJ/ ISFJ	Loss of control over facts and details, impulsiveness, catastrophising	Need to hit bottom, get others to take them seriously, get help with overwhelming detail
ENTP/ ENFP	Withdrawal and depression, obsessiveness, focus on the body	Meditating, getting others to help with physical needs, support, not patronisation

Note: E – Extraversion; S – Sensing; T – Thinking; J – Judging; N – Intuition; I – Introversion; F – Feeling; P – Perceiving.

Change survival guide

Heifetz and Linsky (2002) offer a survival guide that suggests that you need to both manage the environment and yourself to ensure that you survive the change process. Approaches to managing the environment and yourself include the following:

- *Operate in and above the fray:* Observe what's happening to your initiative or project, *as* it's happening. Move back and forth from the dance floor to the balcony, asking, 'What's really going on here?'

- *Court the uncommitted:* The uncommitted but wary are crucial to the success of the initiative. How far are you able to demonstrate how serious you are about making the change? Can you remove people who can't or won't make the required changes? Practise what you preach, and be seen to do it.

- *Cook the conflict:* Keep the heat high enough to motivate your teams and others you need to work with, but low enough to prevent explosions. *Raise the temperature* to make people confront hidden conflicts and other tough issues. Then *lower the heat* to reduce destructive turmoil. Slow the pace of change. Deliver humour, breaks and images of a brighter future.

- *Place the work where it belongs:* Resist resolving conflicts yourself if they are not your conflicts – people will blame *you* for whatever turmoil results. Mobilise *others* to solve problems. Perhaps more important is how you support and manage yourself and prevent yourself from burning out or self-destructing during difficult change.

- *Restrain your desire for control and need for importance:* Order for its own sake prevents organisations from handling contentious issues. And an inflated self-image fosters unhealthy dependence on you.

- *Anchor yourself:* Use a safe place (e.g. a friend's kitchen table) or routine (e.g. a daily walk) to repair any psychological damage and recalibrate your moral compass. Acquire a confidant (*not* an ally from your organisation) who supports you, and not necessarily your initiative. Read challenges and disagreements as reactions to your professional role, not to you personally. You will remain calmer and keep people engaged.

Other processes

Action learning sets: A helpful peer support process is to create an action learning set with others from across the system. These are powerful ways of tapping into the professional expertise and support of others, with a focus on finding a solution to a particular issue. AQuA used these as part of the Discovery Communities discussed earlier, and they have developed so that they exist beyond the life of the programme and participants offer peer coaching to each other.

Mentoring/coaching: Find a supportive mentor, perhaps from a different organisation, or arrange to have a coach who can support you through the implementation process. Consider team coaching, if the dynamics within the team are proving difficult.

Manage expectations: Create a compact with the person who is acting as project sponsor or programme manager in terms of the expectations you have about levels of support – in particular, if there are challenging issues to address or delivery may slip.

Reflection and learning: It is critical to be able to carve out and value time to reflect on how things are going, what has worked well and what you have learned from what has not worked so well. Create 'safe spaces' where you can take yourself apart (and put yourself back together again!). This could be through a coaching relationship, or through more formal supervision approaches. You also need to recognise the emotional labour aspect of what you are doing.

You will probably have your own methods for enabling your own reflective practice, so here we reinforce the need for it, and suggest some frameworks to help think about the importance and the process of reflection when delivering a complex change. One useful approach is restorative supervision, an evidence-based model that has been designed to support the needs of professionals working in roles that demand they have clear thinking and are able to process information quickly and accurately in order to make decisions. The model shows that when professionals undertake complex work they move between anxiety, fear or stress about their work. If they can process these natural feelings about the work, they are able to focus on their own learning needs and development and then they enter a creative, energetic and solution-focused zone (Wallbank 2011).

Reflective debriefing: Reflecting with others (or just yourself) after meetings, or presentations, is a helpful way of gaining peer support, insight and feedback in order to learn from past experience. Figure 4.6 presents a structured cycle for reflective debriefing.

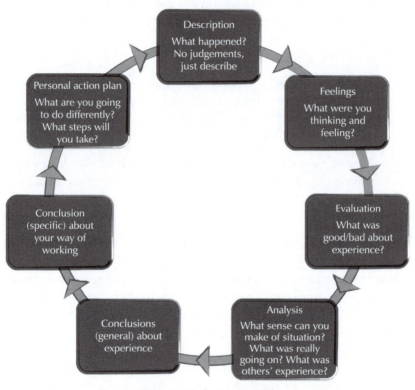

Figure 4.6: Reflective debriefing
Source: Based on Gibbs (1988)

Chapter 5

Managing Change
Processes and People

Chapter 4 took you through the issues relating to leading change. This chapter addresses the means by which change can be managed, so that the process becomes more predictable, and you are more likely to achieve the desired result.

There are, of course, different types of change. Organisational change literature makes a distinction between planned or intentional change, and emergent or spontaneous change. It also makes a distinction between episodic and continuous change, and between transitional and transformational change (Iles and Sutherland 2001). Continuous change is ongoing and evolving and less dramatic in nature and outcome (transitional) – it is sometimes referred to as first order or incremental change. Episodic change can be defined as infrequent and intentional – and may be more dramatic or transformational in nature and outcome. It is sometimes referred to as radical or second order change (Weick and Quinn 1999).

First order, incremental or transactional change is usually about doing existing things better and is seen as normal and a continuous process of improvement and learning. It might involve analysing data, understanding different perspectives such as those of staff and service users, mapping processes and identifying and trying out potential improvements. The Plan, Do, Study, Act (PDSA) cycle is now used quite commonly within public sector organisations as part of a continual process of learning and improvement (see Chapter 6).

Second order, radical or transformational change is about doing things fundamentally differently. It is often resisted initially and needs to be 'sold' to people. It takes longer to implement and embed. It is this kind of change that we focus on in this chapter. We explore its implications by considering the management of those processes required for such change and the management of people affected by this kind of change.

In this chapter we therefore cover the following topics under the two broad themes of managing processes and managing stakeholders:

- How can we keep change on track?

- What approaches will build change for the future?

- Who are the key stakeholders and what is their influence?

- How can we positively support staff in the change process?

- What enables good communication?

How can we keep change on track?

A structured process to managing change, for example a recognised project management approach such as PRINCE2,[1] can bring certain benefits. It allows for greater control over proceedings, determines responsibilities and accountabilities between people, measures progress, keeps things on track, provides a framework for decisions to be made and keeps an eye on the resources being used to make the change happen. Good project management techniques also mean that the effectiveness of the change, or improvement, is actively evaluated and lessons are learned. But whatever approach you take to managing the change, you should not be a slave to a theoretical manual. Formal processes should be introduced as a means to an end and not as an end in themselves. Any approach you take to manage the change should be proportionate to the task, and not be so prescriptive as to prevent flexible and creative solutions.

Agile project management is a concept that is gaining increasing currency – it is an approach to project management that retains a sense of control but that also allows for more flexibility. As an approach, it moves away from the 'command and control' style of a project manager, who directs the work of their team and tells people what to do, to an environment where the end product or output is developed incrementally and iteratively by all members of the team. In the business environment this would require close collaboration with the end user or customer; in the world of health and social care this might mean that change is co-produced with service users or patients.

---

1   PRINCE2 (an acronym for PRojects IN Controlled Environments) is a process-based method for effective project management. Used extensively by the UK government, PRINCE2 is also widely recognised and used in the private sector, both in the UK and internationally. See https://www.prince2.com/uk/what-is-prince2

Research suggests that change is most likely to be successful when there are simple and clear goals for change, when there is a strong fit between what you are trying to do and local policy and priorities, and when changes take account of local circumstances. Change is also more likely to be successful when leaders are supportive, there is a culture in the organisation that supports change and learning, and there are good inter-agency networks and relationships. It is often suggested that a change initiative is most effective when there is a respected clinical champion and good working relationships between clinicians and managers, and managers and staff are prepared to take calculated risks.

There are a number of models that suggest what steps need to be taken to make change happen successfully. One of the best known is Kotter's '8-Step Change Model' (Kotter 1996). This advises those leading change that the first step to take is to create a sense of urgency – that change has to happen because the current way of doing things is no longer satisfactory, commonly also called 'the burning platform' in cases where the status quo is seen as particularly undesirable. Kotter's model suggests that you need buy-in to the change from at least 75 per cent of your staff at this first stage. This enables you to move to the next stage – forming a powerful coalition of visible support from key people. The next step is to create a simple, values-driven vision for change that is communicated clearly through actions and words. Obstacles to change should be tackled quickly, and short-term achievable goals – often called 'quick wins' – should be evident to build momentum and confidence. However, Kotter urges you not to become complacent and to work to build and sustain change before it is embedded in the culture of the organisation – which is the final stage.

Case example 5.1: Use of Kotter's '8-Step Change Model'

The Advancing Quality Alliance's (AQuA) regional integrated care Discovery Community was created to translate integrated care theory into practice at scale, and to test ways to address the system enablers of integrated care in North West England.

Nineteen health and social care economies participated in the Discovery Community, and Kotter's 8-Step Change Model was used as a framework in conjunction with large-scale change theories. These kinds of models were found to be useful in helping participants who might desire a more directive approach in change management.

What does this case example tell us?

» Even if the change programme you are working with is quite exploratory in nature, many people will find comfort in having some model or framework to work through and relate their experiences to.

» The ability to conceptualise the change process by these means can be a powerful way of engaging people and helping them to understand where they and the organisation are at various time points on the change journey.

It is argued that successful change requires action at four levels (Ferlie and Shortell 2001):

• the whole system (for integrated care contexts this will mean across all the organisations involved in integrated service delivery)

• at the level of each organisation within the system

• at the level of the team, department or service

• and finally, at the individual level.

The change required may vary in scale, so that change at the system level may be small, perhaps just a change of policy or paperwork to reflect new procedures, the impact of which is felt most significantly at the individual practitioner level. Whatever the scale of change for each, it is helpful to think about what needs to happen at these four levels.

It is also worth noting that a change perhaps at the department or team level may be part of a much bigger change programme across the whole organisation or system. In this situation, there may be a whole group of change projects that in combination have a single, overarching objective – this structure is known as a 'programme' of activity. Managing the group of projects or changes to achieve this overarching objective is called 'programme management'. Knowing whether the change you are planning or managing is part of a wider programme of activity for a shared purpose, or a stand-alone activity, is important. This will help you to understand what processes you might need to follow, and how your actions might affect the actions of others and the successful delivery of the overarching objective. Figure 5.1 shows how a change to services might fit into a programme structure.

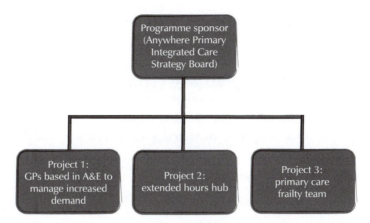

Figure 5.1: Programme structure

Some project management techniques can be particularly helpful in making sure that the change keeps on track. If you are managing the change, you will need to be thinking about all of the following activities, making sure that they are being undertaken by someone in the team, if not by you:

- *Plan, design and schedule:* Decide what needs to happen and when by, and how you will make sure things are happening as they should.

- *Manage resources:* Determine what skills you need to help you achieve your objective and how you can access these skills, and how much it will cost to make the change and where the budget will come from.

- *Define tasks and outputs required:* Break down the required change into a series of tasks that can be articulated, with a clear picture of what output that task should achieve, and assign someone to undertake these tasks on your behalf.

- *Assess, review and report on progress:* Check that things are happening as they should, and keep people informed of progress.

- *Handle issues and take appropriate action:* If things aren't going to plan, you will be responsible for deciding what needs to happen to bring things back on track and making sure that corrective action is taken.

- *Act as central point of contact between all stakeholders:* You will be the person that holds all the threads of the change together and should have an overview of what is happening at all times.

- *Communicate:* You will be responsible for ensuring everyone knows what's happening and why, who will be affected and when, and where the change will happen and how it will happen.

Table 5.1 sets out some terminology that you may come across when managing a change or a project. It is useful to know these terms and how they fit into an overall scheme of activity, as other people in your own organisation or other organisations in the system might be using them.

Table 5.1: Project management terminology

Term	What it includes and how it is used
Project mandate	Authority to proceed
Project brief	Background – why are we doing this? Definitions – objectives, scope, outputs What will outputs look like? Major risks What will happen if the project is not undertaken?
Project plan	Timescales by when things should happen and key decision points
Outline business case	How does the change support the organisational strategy? What are the expected benefits? What are the costs of achieving these?
Risk register	Assessing risk in terms of likelihood, impact and distance away Assigning responsibility for undertaking mitigating actions
Project initiation document (PID)	This is often the key document for a project and includes elements from the project brief, business case, project plan and risk register It describes the project controls in place such as how progress is reported, how costs are managed and how quality is assured It includes the communication plan – who is communicated with, when, why and how
Benefits plan	Describes what benefits are expected from the change process and when these should be realised

As a minimum it is always worth having a document such as a project brief that sets out clearly what you are trying to do, and why, and how things will work once the change has happened. This document might include the activities that have to happen in order to make the change work, when these will happen by, and who is responsible for undertaking them. It might also be important to make a clear statement about who has authorised or approved this change to happen. The document should be reviewed regularly, so that if something changes – perhaps a new national policy is introduced that will change working practices, or organisations merge, or new organisations are created – you can use this document to think through what impact this change will have on what you are trying to do, and whether you need to change what you are doing to respond.

Below is an example of the use of dashboards as a mechanism by which an integrated care change programme is monitored.

Case example 5.2: North West London (NWL) whole systems integrated care pioneer dashboard

NWL decided to set up a mechanism by which outcomes could be measured and tracked. At the outset, it was decided to use a small number of important metrics to capture and monitor to reduce the difficulty of collecting data, and to make it easier to review more frequently and quickly. There was a pragmatic trade-off between metrics that capture important issues but are complicated to collect, and metrics that would allow more reliable data collection. A visualisation dashboard was therefore determined as the best way by which a range of people could see quickly and clearly how progress matched aspirations for the change.

What does this case example tell us?

Best practice was followed in designing the dashboard so that the most important metrics were placed side-by-side on a single page, colour and visuals were used to quickly draw attention to where it was needed, and it was capable of being updated and reviewed frequently.

An illustrative example of such a dashboard is given in Figure 5.2.

Domain	Metric	Q1	Q2	Q3	Q4
Quality of care	• Listening carefully?	58%	70%	73%	85%
	• Given enough time?	61%	72%	70%	83%
	• Understanding how health needs affect life?	64%	75%	76%	86%
Care organisation	• Who is in charge?	48%	58%	60%	70%
	• How to contact?	45%	53%	57%	65%
	• Well organised?	55%	64%	65%	78%
Care planning	• Agreed a care plan?	52%	57%	63%	67%
	• Involved in plan?	43%	55%	62%	65%
	• Holds a copy?	35%	42%	55%	62%

Figure 5.2: An example of a dashboard

What approaches will build change for the future?

Whatever approach you take to managing the change process, it is important to recognise the point at which the change has happened, and that you are now operating in the 'new' world. This is the point at which any new processes and procedures must be embedded in the way the organisation works, and seen as 'the way we do things around here', rather than as a parallel way of operating. It is not uncommon for a change process to be managed as a project and for it never to be 'handed over' or mainstreamed. If this happens, it means that the change is probably unsustainable from both a financial point of view and in terms of changing practices and behaviour.

It is also important to think about what you have learned from the experience of going through the change process, and to try and extract the lessons to reflect on yourself and to share with others. Remember, it is just as valuable to reflect on what didn't work so well as what did. To be able to share the learning effectively, it is useful to organise an event that allows people to talk openly about their experiences of the change process and to capture these reflections. The timing of this will need to ensure that recall is not problematic but that the change has had time to bed down and its impact can be properly assessed. If the change process is drawn out, it might be useful to think about interim learning opportunities, so that important issues aren't forgotten 'in the mists of time'. You might find it helpful during the change process to keep a list of ideas that occur to you as to how you might have gone about doing something differently or why you would do something exactly the same way again. This doesn't have to be a lengthy formal document but could take the form of a scrapbook with post-it notes, or a white board with bullet points – anything to jog the memory when you come to think about how things went and how you would approach something similar again.

If you are committed to the process of organisational learning, the following points are worth bearing in mind:

- Try to encourage people to think not just about what they have learned, or what their own organisation has learned, but what the process of going through the change has meant for the system as a whole.

- You will need some information and data to look at and analyse to help the review process – this might be in the form of quantitative or qualitative data – but it is worth thinking at the outset of a change process what information might help you reflect on the learning later, and to try to ensure these mechanisms for collecting evidence and experience are put in place.

- Some information may potentially provide a negative view of the change, or of the contribution of particular individuals or teams/departments, so it is important to recognise that people might need some support to be able to review the learning in an objective and dispassionate manner.

- Leading on from this, people should be encouraged to acknowledge when things are not working as soon as possible, so that remedial action can be taken, and the situation does not worsen. This will mean ensuring that people feel comfortable raising problems and concerns, and are assured that something will happen as a result of them doing so.

- Constructive challenge is an important part of organisation life and learning, and should be encouraged.

- Productive organisational learning needs to be nurtured – it needs time, focus and skilled facilitation.

Once you have shared the learning amongst your own team, or within your own organisation, you might want to think about spreading your knowledge more widely. However, it has long been recognised that the spread of innovation in the NHS and social care is slow and sporadic, even though sharing this kind of knowledge is what will ultimately drive quality improvements and more effective ways of working.

The Health Foundation (2014) undertook a review of the evidence on what works in spreading improvement ideas. This piece of work suggests that most of the ways that we usually try to do this are limited, either because we simply don't have the evidence to demonstrate their success over a sustained period of time, or because certain methods may only work well in certain circumstances. However, it does suggest that clinical change champions or opinion leaders are valuable.

But whatever the mechanism, the evidence suggests that a passive approach involving knowledge transfer is less likely to be more effective than a proactive approach involving knowledge exchange. For example, sending information out to people either in printed form or through electronic means such as a website is unlikely to engender behaviour change, though a peer-to-peer session based on benchmarking, challenge and discussion might work more effectively.

The recognition that others are involved in, or might benefit from, your experience of undertaking a change process takes us on nicely to the topic of stakeholders, which we now consider in more detail.

Who are the key stakeholders and what is their influence?

There will be groups of people or individuals affected by the changes you are proposing, and there will be those who will have a view on the change, even if they are not directly affected themselves. The obvious groups are service users and their carers, but commissioners of services, the local community and the media may all be influential in either supporting the change or opposing it. You therefore need strategies to work out who your stakeholders are, what issues they are interested in, and what their level and sphere of influence is likely to be. It might be helpful to draw up a stakeholder map of these.

In the example below, we've drawn up a stakeholder map for a fictitious change about the introduction of an integrated service whereby social workers who specialise in working with people with mental health issues are based in GP practices during normal opening hours in order to provide advice, signposting and initial assessments for people referred to them by their GP or another agency. In this fictitious example, the local practice staff and social workers might be broadly supportive of introducing this service because they can see a need for it, but the GP receptionists might feel they are not well prepared to help some of the people now coming to visit their practice. Service users who might benefit from the service might feel anxious about the stigma of accessing it from within their GP practice, whilst other practice patients might feel concerned about using the practice alongside people who they think might have serious mental health problems. In addition, local residents may feel similarly concerned about a new group of people accessing the GP practice. The local media might be an influential ally to publicise the additional service, but could also support local residents to raise their concerns about the change in people visiting the practice.

The ticks in Table 5.2 show which aspects of the change are of most interest or concern to each group of stakeholders.

Table 5.2: Stakeholders and areas of interest

Stakeholder	Increasing access to services	Changes to previous arrangements	Changes to people using the practice
Service users who might benefit from the new service	✓	✓	
Service users who will not benefit from the new service			✓
GP practice staff	✓	✓	✓
Social workers	✓	✓	
Media	✓		✓
Local residents			✓
Commissioners	✓		

Once you have thought about who might have a vested interest in which issues, you can begin to think about how influential they may be in supporting or opposing the change, and how much focus and energy to give to each group or individual. The matrix in Figure 5.3, using the example given above, shows how groups or individuals can be assessed as having a level of importance to the project in terms of helping or hindering it to achieve its objectives, and what the likely impact of the change will be on them. For those stakeholders who are assessed as being highly important to the success of the project and being the most affected by it, you will need to ensure strong buy-in to what you are trying to do, whilst for those who might be only slightly affected and have little influence on the success of the project, you may just need to keep them informed of progress on a regular basis.

It is worth reviewing your stakeholder maps and influence matrix on a regular basis as events or circumstances may happen that can change the range of topics people are interested in, or the level of influence they have over time.

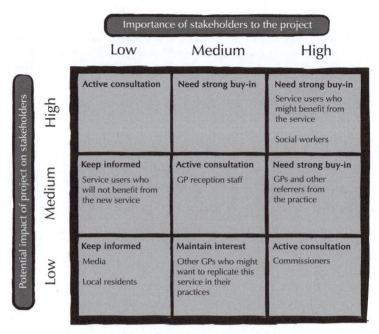

Figure 5.3: Importance and impact of stakeholders

How can we positively support staff in the change process?

It is often said that the hardest part of managing change is convincing staff that change is necessary. Resistance is inevitable and can feel frustrating, but it's worth bearing in mind that resistance from people can also be helpful as it usually shows there are issues that need to be addressed before the change can be made effectively. Helping staff see the need for change requires leadership buy-in and the articulation of a clear vision of the desired future state. It might be necessary to provide some practical support to staff to help them make the necessary changes, to help them through their uncertainties or anxieties, but regardless of the amount of support provided, it is important to recognise that managing change takes time, energy and expertise.

It is suggested that sources of resistance to change can appear at two stages – first, the stage at which the change initiative is formulated, and second, at the stage of implementation (Pardo del Val and Martinez 2003). For example, sources of resistance at the point at which change is formulated might include myopia, so staff do not have a vision of what the future is likely to require; financial, so that the costs of change might seem too heavy to bear; or past experience, so people dwell on past failures and are sceptical that the organisation can succeed this time around. The sources of resistance at the implementation stage might include departmental politics, so one entity might be perceived to be a winner from the change programme, whilst another might be perceived as losing out; embedded routines that are really tough to change; or a lack of necessary capabilities.

It is possible therefore that different strategies and tactics might be required to address resistance to change at different stages of the change process. The following three subsections may help you think more specifically about working with staff through the change process, and how to begin to influence them effectively.

Trust/agreement matrix

In terms of influencing people, it is helpful to think about where to put your energies and what strategies are likely to work for people who may either support you from the outset, are sceptical but prepared to see what happens, and those who oppose you outright. Various models have been developed over time that put people into different categories depending on whether they are in agreement with you or not, and whether they trust and respect you or not. Figure 5.4 provides our own version of these categories.

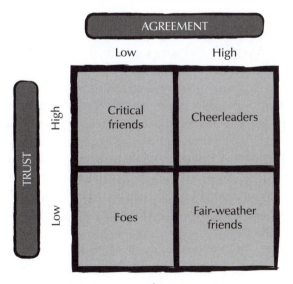

Figure 5.4: Trust/agreement matrix

Your cheerleaders are those you can rely on for full support. You can maintain this support by affirming the importance of the relationship, asking for their advice and encouraging them to advocate on your behalf with others.

A critical friend may be someone who you respect and trust and who respects and trusts you but disagrees with you on this particular issue. These people can offer valuable alternative perspectives, and it might be helpful to proactively seek them out to identify whether their views ought to influence the direction you are taking and if there is any common ground to work from.

A fair-weather friend might be in agreement with you but you might feel they are working from a hidden agenda and may not be trusted to maintain their alignment, especially if things don't always seem to be going according to plan. With these people, you might confirm that you need their support, but acknowledge your concerns, and try to establish clear shared goals that are less likely to be subject to change.

The foe is the greatest challenge, and you might expend a lot of effort and not change people's minds to bring them on board. The best approach may be to keep communication channels open and demonstrate that you are always ready to discuss things, but that you will be taking the course of action you have set out.

Adoption of innovation

We discussed above the importance of sharing knowledge and improvement and how you might think about doing this across departments, teams and organisations. However, it isn't easy for some people to adopt new ideas or to change their ways of doing things.

Some people will seize on new ideas enthusiastically and will want to do things as soon as possible, such as buying the latest gadgets as soon as they come out; others will adopt a more cautious approach and will wait for others to test out the ideas first, or for evidence that they will work to be produced, such as waiting a while until they have read magazine reviews of the latest phone or TV and then deciding to buy; still other colleagues may wilfully hold on to the 'old ways' of doing things even when everyone else has moved on, seemingly taking pride in remaining untouched by 'progress'.

It is perhaps helpful at this point to think about the adoption model (Rogers 2003). The model, which is based on the classic bell curve, classifies people as innovators who are highly motivated people seeking out continual change (it is suggested that only 2.5 per cent of the population are innovators) through to laggards, traditionalists who are reluctant to change even when the evidence to do so is strong (16 per cent of the population). Early adopters follow the innovators – they need a little support but they adopt change quickly and are opinion leaders; the early majority need convincing, but follow when results look positive; whilst the late majority join in when the change becomes accepted practice (see Figure 5.5).

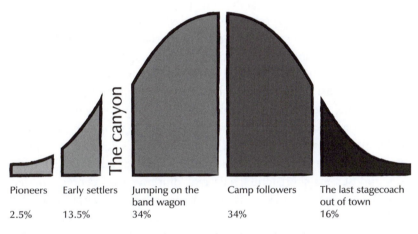

Pioneers	Early settlers	Jumping on the band wagon	Camp followers	The last stagecoach out of town
2.5%	13.5%	34%	34%	16%

Figure 5.5: Adoption of innovation

Recognising how many people are likely to be in each group might help give managers a bit of heart when it looks as though change is taking a long time to happen, or people are being very slow to adopt new ways of working.

Rogers (2003) also suggests that there are five factors that help spread and embed change. The first is that the advantages of the new way of doing things are clear, with evidence to show the change has made an improvement and that benefits go beyond service users; the second is that the change is of low complexity, so that it is easy to understand and publicise; the third is compatibility, so that the change fits with how people work and their values; the fourth is trialability, trying something out without making a full commitment to it; and the fifth is adaptability, so that the change can be adapted to the individual needs of the organisation and of teams.

Managing transitions

Whatever the scale of the change, there will always be a transition phase between the old way of doing things and the new way. When the old way of doing things comes to an end, and before the new way of doing things becomes second nature for people, there will be a 'neutral' phase, when neither the old way, nor the new way, is working fully, and things can feel quite confusing. During this period staff may feel quite anxious and demotivated. It might take longer to get things done and there may be more problems to sort out. This can be frustrating for people who are trying to carry on delivering a high quality service.

Transition requires people to consciously accept the new way of doing things, and this can take time. It is important to talk people through this process by giving them the opportunity to express how they feel, to recognise what they feel they are losing and to articulate what is to be gained. It is also important to acknowledge what was good about the previous state, and how it has been a positive legacy from which to build, as rubbishing what has gone before will only make people feel devalued.

During the transition phase, a number of actions to manage it positively may be important. These might include developing temporary roles and setting short-term goals and objectives, so people can feel there is a sense of progress. It is also important not to overpromise what can be achieved during this period, when productivity is unlikely to be optimal, so keep expectations lowered amongst staff, managers and other stakeholders. Providing some training on teamwork or problem-solving, or having an away-day to review, regroup and reassert, can also be helpful. Good communication and consistent messages are key to the successful navigation of the transition phase. When going through a change, it is important for managers to say what they know, say what they don't know, and to commit to a time to give people more information.

You are likely to find yourself reiterating to people what the purpose of the change is, providing a vision of how the future state will look and feel, providing some more detailed sense of the steps needed to get there, as and when they become known, and reassuring people that they have a role to play in the new vision of how things will be and that their contribution is important to the overall success of the change effort.

As with so much activity relating to change, possessing good communication skills will be crucially important when dealing with all stakeholders, whether staff or external. We have therefore included a final section in this chapter on the topic.

What enables good communication?

Communication is something that we all do every day, and most of us probably think we are effective communicators, so it is worth reflecting on the following maxim: 'The single biggest problem with communication is the illusion that it has taken place.'

So what makes someone a good communicator, or something a good piece of communication? Being a good communicator does not mean, of course, that you have to be a powerful and persuasive public orator, but it does mean that you need to think about the what, why, when, where, who and how of communication carefully. Asking yourself a series of questions as follows should help:

- What is the purpose of the communication? Is it to provide information? Is it to influence people to think, feel or act in a particular way? What will be communicated? Facts and figures? Complex information? Personal stories or case studies? Will you be providing short summary communications, or long and detailed communications?

- When is the best time to communicate? Continuously? Regularly? Only when there is good news? Only when things are not going according to plan? As soon as you know about an issue, a problem or a success, but before any of the detail is known? How often will you need to repeat the same communication?

- Where will the communication be delivered and seen/heard? Will your communication be publically accessible? Does the location of your communication create bias or inequalities of access? Will it be visible to the people you want it to be visible to?

- Who will receive the communication? Will the recipients be policy-makers and professionals, or service users, carers or citizens? Will you need to change the language accordingly? Remove abbreviations or acronyms and jargon? Will you need to simplify the language, or translate materials?

- Who will be communicating? Does the communication need to be made by the most senior person in an organisation for symbolic purposes? Do you need to be the one communicating the information to build trust? Is it better to have an external person communicating to show objectivity? Will a service user communicating create more impact?

- How will you communicate? Do you have any resources to spend on communication activities? Are you communicating face-to-face or by virtual channels? Are you using traditional print media or video? Are you using digital or social media? Are you communicating in the first person, or in the third? Do you need some professional assistance to make your communication have an impact?

Whatever channel you decide is appropriate to use for your communication and whoever your audience is, it is important to ensure that you communicate honestly, accurately and consistently. Research tells us that people forget most of the information they are told verbally within minutes of hearing it, and that the information they do remember is often incorrect. It is therefore important that you provide clear, simple messages that can be repeated. It is also worth thinking about providing people with some record of verbal communications they can refer back to later.

Even though you may be tailoring your communication to different groups of people, such as professionals, service users or policy-makers, these are still not homogeneous groups. Research suggests that people have different preferences for the amount of information they want and when they want it. For example, people can be categorised as 'monitors' or 'blunters' (Miller 1987), whereby monitors want as much information as possible prior to any decisions they have to make and blunters find too much information overwhelming. The terms 'big chunkers' and 'little chunkers' represent the difference between those who just want the 'big picture' information and do not want to be bothered with the detail, and those who want as much detail as possible.

Of course, it will not be possible to get it right for everyone all of the time, but knowing that there are these variations in how people prefer to receive information and communicate is nonetheless helpful in improving your skills. Other practical tips for improving your communication include giving the most important information first; limiting the amount of information provided; personalising or contextualising messages, so people can relate to them; using visual images to provide clarity and help with recall; and creating an environment where people feel able to ask questions and provide comments – after all, communication should be a two-way process.

We have come to the end of this chapter on managing change, and it is now time to turn our attention to evaluating change.

Chapter 6

Evaluating and Reviewing Integration

Evaluating and *reviewing* are often seen as quite different activities. Evaluating is frequently interpreted as a more formal, academic activity that can therefore feel intimidating for those without a formal research background. Common concerns for practice leaders include how to choose between different methodologies, how to summon up the energy and capacity to gather and analyse data, and how to cope with the prospect of ending up with results that are incomplete and uninformative. It may be of little consolation for any non-academics feeling this way, but those with formal research experience also often feel intimidated by such evaluations. Their concerns are not generally to do with technical skills, but rather with how to deal with the complexity of different data systems, alternative views of outcomes and multiple contributing factors. They also commonly worry that the organisations concerned will want a definite answer when one is unlikely to be forthcoming. *Reviewing,* on the other hand, is often viewed as being an organisationally led process that will decide if an initiative is delivering value for the organisation(s) involved. It is seen as a more practically orientated exercise that is perhaps less technically demanding, but can have major implications, as the outcome of a review can be to cease, scale down or adapt what is being provided.

Despite these differences, evaluation and review processes actually have a lot in common. They should both be focused on the outcomes that were expected of the initiative, and seek to objectively identify positive achievements as well as those aspects that have not gone so well. They should engage relevant stakeholders in the process, and draw on relevant and accurate sources of data to gather a full picture of what is going on. They should seek to be a facilitator of future learning and improvement.

They also both share a common hazard of being relegated to the bottom of the 'to do list' because the demands of getting an initiative up and running are so exhausting, or because they are seen as potentially 'dangerous' if the findings are not what was expected. They often emerge only when the service has commenced and changes have already been achieved. However, introducing them at this stage means that baselines are lost, data-gathering mechanisms are not embedded, and the whole process can lose credibility before it even begins.

It is vital, though, that evaluation and review are embedded into the design of an integrated care initiative. The gathering and analysis of data as a support for improvement is recognised as a vital part of achieving and sustaining positive change. Without relevant evidence we will not know what works and what does not, and will therefore be working on the basis of intuition and best guessing. We will struggle to focus our energies and resources on the integration approaches that make the most difference in this context. We will not be able to meaningfully share our learning with others and to save future initiatives time and wasteful activity. The good news is that evaluation and review do not have to be intimidating or overwhelming, that there are straightforward tools and techniques that can be drawn on, and that those without a formal research background can produce findings and relevant learning.

In this chapter we take you through the steps you need to think through to plan and complete a basic evaluation or review of an integrated care initiative. As ever this is a start, and not the finish, and we would encourage any of you with an interest to look more into evaluation methodologies and the tools that can support them. Building on the common interpretations given above and the intended audience of the book, we describe this process as an 'evaluative review', an organisational-generated process that is designed to explore what the integrated initiative has achieved and how its impacts can be improved.

In this chapter we cover the following:

- What are the key issues before getting started on an evaluative review?

- What methods will help you to understand 'process' and 'benefits'?

- How can you learn from and share your findings?

What are the key issues before getting started on an evaluative review?

In Chapter 2 we discussed the importance of mapping the integrated care initiative in order to understand what outcomes will be delivered and how these will be achieved. We will therefore assume that this mapping has been completed. Before beginning the review, there are a number of key practical issues that need to be sorted. Some of these can only be fully addressed when you know the details of what it will entail, but it is important to begin thinking about them in advance, as they will also influence the scale and type of the exercise. Not taking the time to consider and respond to these issues runs the risk that data will be gathered that is not robust or relevant, or that key outcomes and interests are not responded to adequately. As well as not providing the insights and learning that would be hoped for, a poorly planned and implemented review can be frustrating to all concerned. This can, in turn, lead to a loss of goodwill and waste of resources that means that others may not participate in such evaluation and review activity in the future.

Why are you undertaking the evaluative review?

The key aim of such a process is attempting to understand if an intervention has achieved its expected purpose. Beyond this core aim, evaluative reviews may be required to respond to a wide variety of motivations and interests. The range of purposes that may be expected are outlined in Table 6.1. It is possible to achieve multiple purposes from the same process, but these may need different types of data and methods that can, in turn, expand the time and resources beyond the budget and timescales allowed. Prioritising which purposes will be the most important is therefore crucial, and this will require engaging with your stakeholders (see the section on stakeholder maps in Chapter 5) to develop a common set of expectations. Without these there is a danger that the findings will not be of relevance or interest or have the intended impact.

Table 6.1: Common purposes of evaluative reviews

Purpose	Objective
Accountability	To demonstrate to stakeholders that the integrated care initiative has fulfilled the expected requirements
Sustainability	To secure or maintain the funding and resources necessary to sustain the integrated care initiative

cont.

Purpose	Objective
Roll-out	To convince stakeholders that the integrated care initiative should be rolled out into other services and localities
Improvement	To provide feedback that can be used to further improve the integrated care initiative
Social value	To identify the wider value of the integrated care initiative beyond those immediately recognised by the participants and staff
Learning	To gather experiences of what worked (and what did not) in this aspect of integrated care for sharing with interested parties (including through professional or academic journals)
Marketing	To use as a means to promote the work of the integrated care initiative and its contributing partners

What is the focus of your evaluative review?

Establishing the purpose(s) of the evaluative review will then help to inform its focus. For example, if the main purpose is to establish if the funding provided was an efficient means to produce the expected benefits, then the focus will be a *summative* assessment of the outcomes and costs. If, however, the main purpose is to understand the learning to date to improve the future working of the integrated care initiative, then the evaluative review will have a *formative* focus on the experiences of the individuals involved (see Case examples 6.1 and 6.2). The different focuses are commonly themed under the terms 'process', 'impact' and 'economic'. Once again, it is possible for a single evaluation to cover all of these different focuses with the correct design and sufficient resources:

- *Process:* The focus is on how an integrated care initiative has been developed and implemented. Issues of interest often include communication within and outside the initiative, coordination of service user care and support, managing the change and addressing resistance, oversights and incentives, and training and development (the resources and activities elements of the mapping carried out in Chapter 2).

- *Impact:* The focus is on the outcomes of an integrated initiative for service users, families and/or the overall health of the population (mirroring the outcomes in Chapter 2). The benefits (or otherwise) for professionals and practitioners are also often considered. To formally demonstrate 'impact', the extent to which these outcomes have been achieved has to be compared with what would have happened without the integrated care initiative being in place. This is commonly called 'the counterfactual'.

- *Economic:* The focus is on the 'value for money' of the integrated care initiative. This can include what it costs (i.e. what resources are required to plan and deliver the initiative) and its wider financial consequences (commonly on resource usage in other parts of the system). If the focus is just on 'what it costs', this is described as a 'cost-effectiveness analysis', but if the focus is on the wider impacts, it is termed a 'cost benefit analysis'.

Case example 6.1: Aims and objectives of OPM's evaluation of the Advancing Quality Alliance (AQuA)

The aims of the evaluation were to provide an understanding of how the model and elements of the programme supported large-scale system change, and to explore the transferability of the model to other system-level reforms.

Key objectives were to:

» understand how the different elements of the programme supported large-scale change – in particular, the framework of the master classes and workshops and the additional tailored and bespoke support

» demonstrate the impact of the programme in supporting individuals and teams to implement large-scale system change, including reviewing the measures being used by local teams to assess success, as well as the impact of the programme on leadership capacity and capability within partnership teams

» explore the contextual factors and other activities/strategic priorities that impact on engagement and progress with the programme at an economy level

» explore the factors that enable or impede effective engagement and implementation of the learning

» explore the feasibility and potential benefits of providing a suite of offers for individuals and teams to increase the breadth and depth of the learning experience

» test the applicability of the programme framework and delivery model for other programmes of system-level change and reform, including the public health and wellbeing agenda, as a future potential membership and customer offer.

What does this case example tell us?

» This evaluation had a major focus on the process of change and how the programme design worked in practice.

» It considered impacts on individuals and teams, and the potential application of the learning for future programmes.

Source: OPM (2015)

Case example 6.2: Economic evaluation of the Partnerships for Older People Programme (POPP)

Under POPP, 29 projects were funded, which between them operated a total of 146 core interventions. The Personal Social Services Research Unit (PSSRU) in London completed a large-scale national evaluation. The Nuffield Trust was then asked to complete a more focused evaluation of a small, but carefully selected, set of eight POPP interventions. They were asked to examine in detail whether these interventions had been successful in avoiding emergency admissions to hospital. Through the use of anonymised data linkage, the Nuffield Trust was able to construct matched control groups for the eight POPP interventions. These control groups matched the intervention groups very well in terms of a wide range of characteristics, including age, sex, area-level deprivation, medical diagnoses, predicted risk of hospital admission (PARR scores – patients at risk of readmission) and prior healthcare use. Compared with some alternative evaluation approaches, this allowed them to measure more precisely the impact of the interventions on hospital use.

What does this case example tell us?

» The evaluation was focused on the economic impact of the interventions, and, in particular, the effects on hospital admissions.

» Through matching the population targeted by the intervention with other comparable populations, the evaluation was able to explore the counterfactual.

Source: Steventon et al. (2011)

What resources are available to support the evaluative review?

In an ideal world, each integrated care initiative would be able to access external evaluation support. This is on the basis that it fosters greater independence and objectivity to the research that can make the findings seem more robust to external stakeholders. It also brings in additional capacity so that busy managers and practitioners do not have to try and do evaluation on top of their day jobs. There are potential drawbacks, though. If there is not a good understanding between the external evaluation team and the integrated care initiative, then the evaluators may focus on what they think is important rather than what the service needs to prioritise. Having external researchers spending time within the service can feel disruptive and distracting, particularly if their purpose has not been fully explained and their engagement insufficiently planned. It can also result in staff members not owning the findings if they believe that the external researchers did not grasp how the service worked and the benefits it could deliver. Usually, though, the main issue regarding the enlistment of external support is the issue of obtaining funding for their time. That said, it is possible, with funding sometimes being provided by the organisations and partnerships that oversee the integrated care initiative, and there are also occasional grants available from local public sector or charitable bodies. It can also be that a local university has been awarded a separate research grant and is looking for a case study site to undertake this research.

This chapter is written on the basis that there is no funding to pay for an external evaluation team. There are, though, still a number of potential options for drawing in additional capacity to support and improve the evaluation process. Staff members working within the integrated care initiative may have an interest in research and be looking for the opportunity to undertake research as part of their professional development. This could be as part of an evaluation team or more individual 'practitioner-led research' (see Case example 6.3). This is research completed by practitioners, rather than university-based researchers; that focus on the practice of the practitioner and/or their peers; that are short term and of a small scale; and that are not linked to a larger research programme.

Case example 6.3: Practitioner-led research

Practitioner-led research is usually carried out alone, but in this case, two practitioners working in partnership carried it out – a social worker from the local authority and a carers support worker from the third sector. They wanted to explore how different approaches to working with carers (a statutory sector carers assessment and a voluntary sector outcomes-focused approach) would contribute to the outcomes experienced by carers.

Data gathering included semi-structured focus groups with carers and practitioners, and document analysis of the blank and completed tools used by each organisation. Beyond the important insights into the impact of these practices on carers, the two practitioners also reflected on their own experiences of researching in this way. They found undertaking the work together enabled them to understand better each other's frames of reference and facilitated better communication. It provided an opportunity for personal development, and led to increased confidence in their individual and joint knowledge. The findings were presented to both organisations, and this led to a redesign of pathways and assessment tools. They also experienced difficulties in relation to sharing information between the organisations.

What does this case example tell us?

» This research highlights that small-scale projects completed by individual practitioners can provide meaningful insights.

» Through their practical focus the findings were relevant for the organisation and facilitated improvements in the experience of service users.

» The project also led to personal development for the practitioners concerned.

Source: Gamiz and Tsegai (2014)

Alongside staff members working in the service there may be other staff members within organisations who are undertaking university degrees and who are looking to complete their research as part of their Master's dissertations, and for whom a case study site would provide excellent data. Twinning up with another service can be a way of agreeing to 'swap' staff members to undertake observations and interviews. This can provide a 'fresh pair of eyes' that can help with objectivity and enable everyday practice to be seen in a different way. It can also lead to the staff members concerned taking back ideas and insights into their own services, and demonstrate to them the potential of more effective integration. Similarly, drawing on volunteer user-researchers can also add much to an evaluation (see Case example 6.4). Such volunteers need to be properly supported through training and mentoring, and any expenses should be met. Their aspirations from participating should also be discussed and responded to, so that they directly benefit from the experience.

Case example 6.4: Example of a service user-researcher

This study sought to investigate the information, advice and support needs of older people experiencing a transition between services. This included discharge out of hospital and into services for people with dementia. The project followed a 'participative action research methodology', with service users and carers from each area being recruited, trained and supported to participate as co-researchers. Working with academic project team members, co-researchers jointly conducted two waves of in-depth interviews to explore the experience of care transitions from a user/carer perspective.

Information about the study and the opportunity to participate was circulated through local voluntary sector networks and in person by research leads at older people's groups and meetings. People interested in becoming co-researchers were asked to fill out a short application form, and took part in a face-to-face or telephone interview. The interview allowed research leads to establish people's eligibility and suitability for the role, as well as giving applicants the opportunity to find out more about what being a co-researcher would entail.

A training programme was designed and delivered in a number of half-day sessions over the duration of the study. The training fulfilled three main purposes:

>> *skills development*, enabling co-researchers to learn about the project and to develop or refresh the skills needed for data collection, analysis and presentation

>> *co-design*, creating opportunities for research leads and co-researchers to shape the research process and outcomes together

>> *team building*, bringing the team together to help build relationships and trust, and to foster mutual support.

At the end of the project the co-researchers and academics reflected on the participatory approach. In general this was seen to have been positive in terms of recruitment (co-researchers helped to identify potential forums and indeed individuals), content (participants seemed to feel more at ease and willing to share their experiences) and dissemination (co-researchers were involved in sharing the learning direct with professionals and service user representative groups). The co-researchers had all enjoyed being part of the research, and attributed much of the success of the study to the enthusiasm and competence of the academic leads.

What does this case example tell us?

» This study highlights that service users and carers can positively contribute to all aspects of the evaluation process.

» Meaningful engagement of service users and carers requires planning and support (in line with the engagement and involvement discussions in Chapter 3).

» If done well, the involvement has positive benefits for service users and carers as well as the evaluation.

Source: Ellins et al. (2012)

What are the ethics of your evaluative review?

'Ethics' in this context is sometimes interpreted as the formal ethical review processes that are required by research projects. These arrangements will vary, depending on the country, sector and organisation in which the evaluative review is taking place. There is, though, commonly a distinction between an 'ethics committee' (a formal body that passes judgement on the ethics of individual research projects) and 'research governance' (a broader set of regulations, principles and standards of good practice that exist to achieve, and continuously improve, research quality). In many cases an evaluative review may not require formal approval from an ethics committee, as the level of risk to participants will be relatively low. However, it will still need to comply with the expected research governance processes, and this may require consultation with an organisational committee or function. Whatever the required process, it is important that the related issues are properly considered, as such 'principles that guide conduct' are central both to good evaluative work and the everyday practice of practitioners and professionals.

Whilst the nuances of ethics vary slightly between these professions and sectors, they are based around the key principles of autonomy (respect for individuals), non-maleficence (not doing harm), beneficence (trying to do good) and justice (treating people fairly) (Woolham 2011). Whilst some reviews could only involve anonymised datasets and so do not have any ethical issues, most will involve the active participation of people and/or sensitive personal data, and therefore have the potential at least to breach someone's privacy or cause them distress.

The main ethical issues can be practically translated into a number of elements that should be thought through before proceeding:

- *Consent:* If people are to participate in a review, either through directly communicating through, say, an interview or survey, being observed or providing recognisable data, they should be given the opportunity to consent to this participation.

- *Capacity:* Key to consenting to participation is an individual's capacity to make such a decision. Capacity means that they understand what is being asked of them, they can weigh up the pros and cons, and then communicate this decision. In addition to good practice expectations are legal requirements regarding the engagement of people who may not have capacity within research projects.

- *Withdrawal:* Participants who agree to take part should then have the option to subsequently withdraw their consent, with no implications for their care and support. This must be made clear before the review begins to avoid people becoming anxious as to what the implications would be. This is as true for staff members as for service users and family carers.

- *Confidentiality:* In general it is good practice for people's identity to be withheld to avoid any repercussions that could arise from unpopular views or from them feeling reluctant to share these due to such concerns. Realistically it is not always possible to do so when numbers of participants are low (e.g. there may only be one occupational therapist!). In such cases it is vital that participants understand how the data will be presented so that they can then make an informed decision.

- *Benefits and harms:* The potential *risks* of an evaluative review to potential participants should be mapped out. This will both enable relevant safeguards to be put in place, and for participants to be fully informed. The *benefits* should also be articulated to ensure that a balanced perspective is provided.

It is clear that the key to good ethical practice in relation to such work is being able to communicate with potential participants. This is often achieved through providing an information sheet or similar, with the decision made by the potential participant then being recorded through their signature or other means. Such information needs to be adapted to the communication style of the participant, including non-written and accessible formats.

What methods will help you to understand 'process' and 'benefits'?

Having established the purpose of the evaluation, secured the necessary resources and considered the ethical issues, you are now ready to plan to gather and analyse relevant data. In this section we consider common methods that are applied within the evaluative review of integrated care initiatives.

Before getting into the detail it is worth pausing for a moment to reflect on some broader issues of knowledge and research that often arise within integrated settings. These relate to the underlying 'paradigms' (or ways of seeing the world) that are commonly adopted by different professions and their organisations. To paint a very simple picture, many healthcare professions come from a 'positivist' paradigm, whereas those from a social science base come from a 'constructivist' paradigm (see Table 6.2 for their key characteristics). These assumptions about the world and knowledge are important in relation to evaluative review as they shape the type of evidence that we see as credible. This, in turn, shapes the methods that we see as worthwhile. This difference may manifest itself through some stakeholders not being convinced about qualitative methods and the small samples that they often entail, or others seeing quantitative surveys as having too narrow and simplistic a focus. These debates are being played out within formal research regarding integration, so you are not alone in experiencing such frustration.

Table 6.2: Key elements of 'positivist' and 'constructivist' paradigms

Paradigm aspect	Positivist	Constructivist
What is reality?	There is an overall truth about how the real world operates	Reality is not one thing, but is socially constructed in the minds of individuals and groups
What is the purpose of the research?	Research should seek to establish what this truth is	Research should seek to capture these different perspectives
How does the research interact with reality?	Research should be objective and separate to the reality being studied and should not interfere with it	Research will interact with the subjects of the study and therefore shape and be shaped by it
What is the starting point for the research?	Research begins with a hypothesis that is then investigated to prove/disprove	Research seeks to gain understanding through identifying and building on themes
Classic research designs	Randomised control trials Quasi-experimental design	Ethnographic study Action research Case studies

The methods that are used within the two traditions are sometimes also seen as being split between 'quantitative' (positivism) and 'qualitative' (constructivism). Whilst there is a degree of truth in this, it is a lazy distinction, as there are many examples of a variety of methods being deployed within each paradigm. Mixed methods studies, that is, those that incorporate different sources of data and therefore the means to gather these, are also increasingly deployed. These draw on a 'realist' or 'pragmatic' view of knowledge and the world. Mixed methods can provide a richer picture, and the opportunity to compare and contrast the implications that are being suggested by different datasets (in research terminology, 'to triangulate'). For evaluative reviews we would suggest a pragmatic approach that builds on the 'mapping' of the integrated care initiative completed at the outset and uses the relevant methods to explore the relevant aspects of this. Whilst there is clearly an exotic range of methods that could be considered, in practice, most such evaluations and reviews draw on a number of key ones. These methods are summarised in Table 6.3, with some hints as to their use in practice (we would, of course, recommend that you also consult wider research resources).

Table 6.3: Common methods in an evaluative review

Method	Good for...	Be aware of...
Interviews	Exploring participants' views and experiences in some depth Having the flexibility to respond to the emerging themes and what seems to be important to participants Involving participants who may have difficulty in written communication	The balance between structured questions and the opportunity for participants to raise issues from their own perspective Interviews are a time-intensive means to gather data, particularly if you add in transcribing The participant should be doing most of the talking The interviewer can lead the participant to prioritise certain issues or views
Focus groups	Gathering qualitative data from a number of participants at the same time Generating a range of views and interactions between these Involving participants who may have difficulty in written communication	The influence of group dynamics leading to some participants not being willing to share their views of being influenced It is difficult to explore issues in any depth The skills needed to successfully moderate a group (includes ensuring the group covers the topics and that behaviour between participants is acceptable)
Observations	Rather than relying on what people think they do or inferences from secondary datasets, it is possible to witness what actually happens in practice Getting an initial feel for a service and the potential issues for further exploration Picking up on physical artefacts that can demonstrate aspects of organisational culture	The presence of the observer is likely to influence how the participants behave It can be very time-consuming and there may be periods when not much is happening of interest or relevance The balance between 'informal observation' in which there is freedom to decide what is relevant and worthy of recording, and 'structured observation' which uses fixed schedules of predetermined aspects The degree of interaction the observer will have with participants (and when they may need to step out of role, e.g. in situations of risk or unsafe practice)

Surveys	Gaining views from a large number of people on a small number of issues and/or in limited depth Can be easy to combine responses from a large number of respondents Giving participants the opportunity for anonymous comments (if designed in this way)	Surveys can be administered by interviewers, post, telephone or online The questions should be piloted before the survey is launched to check how people understand the wording and the range of responses Response rates are often low, and those with a burning issue may be more likely to reply, which can influence results They may seem easy to administer, but surveys require considerable planning and implementation to provide good insights
Secondary data analysis	Providing longitudinal quantitative data on the performance of a service including economic aspects If existing record systems can provide the necessary data, this avoids duplication of effort	There is a risk that there is a lot of data but it does not provide any insights into the areas of interest The robustness of the data and any bias or limitations must be recognised
Docu-mentary analysis	Reviewing the initial context, assumptions, planning and expected outcomes of a service Tracking how plans have changed over time – participants will often subsume the current arrangements and forget what previous plans entailed	Documents are produced for a purpose and audience that will therefore shape what they include and how they are interpreted As well as the information the author meant to convey, there will be other insights into how this is presented and what is not included Being clear about the sample of documents and the themes to be explored avoids time being used inefficiently through reading text with no purpose Written documents are not the only form of documentary evidence – websites, Twitter feeds and video formats may also be available

Sources: From practice experience and Robson (2002)

Case examples 6.5 and 6.6 describe two evaluations of integrated care initiatives which combine different methods in their design.

Case example 6.5: Evaluation of Life After Stroke

The Life After Stroke service was developed by the Stroke Association to provide support to stroke survivors when they were discharged from hospital. It highlighted that five types of support should be offered – information and advice, prevention, communication support, reablement and inclusion, and carer support. The national model was incorporated within an existing scheme provided by the local branch, and received funding from health and social care commissioners. Key to local implementation was a number of coordinator posts that took on lead roles such as for employment and shared responsibility for prevention and carer support.

The evaluation used mixed quantitative and qualitative methods, including:

» *documentary analysis*, such as national policy and guidance date reports, commissioning contracts and job descriptions

» *secondary data analysis* of national Stroke Association impact surveys, management reports and a computerised care management system

» *focus groups* held on three occasions with the stroke service coordinators

» a *survey* developed from the national stroke survey and administered at three points of time

» *interviews* completed with stroke survivors, carers and wider stakeholders from the statutory and community sectors.

What does this case example tell us?

» In this evaluation both qualitative and quantitative methods were used to understand the impacts and the process of the service.

» The evaluators used existing datasets, adapted previous survey instruments, and drew up bespoke interview schedules.

» The final report brought together all of these sources and types of data to provide a rich picture.

Source: Jenkins, Brigden and King (2013)

Case example 6.6: Evaluation of Integrated Care in Norfolk (ICN)

The ICN programme involved a mixed methods design to explore impacts in relation to patients, staff and service delivery:

» *Patients*: The multi-disciplinary teams identified 20 patients who had had ICN interventions. Following introductory letters, ten patients agreed to be interviewed on their views and experiences of the service. A semi-structured questionnaire was designed with each question tracking directly to project objectives and patient pledges. Interviews were conducted in the patient's home on a face-to-face basis with two interviewers. Questionnaire responses were analysed using themed content analysis, and were validated with the multi-disciplinary teams and patient records. By August 2011, a total of 845 patients had been recorded on the ICN database as having had assessments and/or interventions.

» *Staff:* A semi-structured questionnaire was designed for individual completion online, for interviews and to guide a collective discussion in focus groups. The questions were mapped to project objectives, and staff were invited to discuss changes to their practice and the service, to express their level of satisfaction and to give their views on the process.

» *Service changes:* In order to assess the impact of changing practice on the way that services were utilised, a data analysis of activity based on practice populations was undertaken, and compared to the rest of Norfolk. A performance dashboard was developed that linked data from organisational sources: NHS Norfolk Hospital Episode Statistics and Secondary Uses Service data, Social Services National Social Services Measures, and local GP practice records.

What does this case example tell us?

» This evaluation highlights how qualitative and quantitative methods can be used to complement each other – for example, the findings of the staff surveys were explored in more depth in the focus groups.

» The evaluation also developed a dashboard that would have potential uses within the operational delivery of the programme.

Source: Tucker and Burgis (2012)

In addition to these general methods are established research 'instruments' that have been developed to measure aspects of integration and integrated care (see below). These are worth considering, as if formally 'validated', they will provide more robust and comparable data than a locally designed instrument. On the negative side, they may not always have the exact focus that is of interest or may miss out key aspects.

Development Model for Integrated Care (DMIC)

The DMIC (Minkman, Ahaus and Huijsman 2009) provides a holistic perspective and is targeted at service delivery. It was originally developed in the Netherlands, but is now being used in North America and elsewhere in Europe, and has been deployed within a range of integrated care services including community mental health and older people's services, cardiology and neurology. The DMIC identifies nine dimensions that are key to integrated care. These dimensions (or clusters) are further broken down into activities (or elements) through which these can be realised in practice (see Figure 6.1). The model also recognises that there are stages in the development of an integrated care service, and that the dimensions will be gradually introduced during implementation. The stages are *Stage 1: Initiative and design, Stage 2: Experiment and execution, Stage 3: Expansion and monitoring,* and *Stage 4: Consolidation and transformation.*

The DMIC can be administered through surveys and as the basis for interviews and focus group discussions. It can be helpful at all stages of the development and implementation of an inter-professional team, from initially deciding if the context will be supportive of such a team being introduced, to reviewing progress in achieving the expected impacts and supporting team processes.

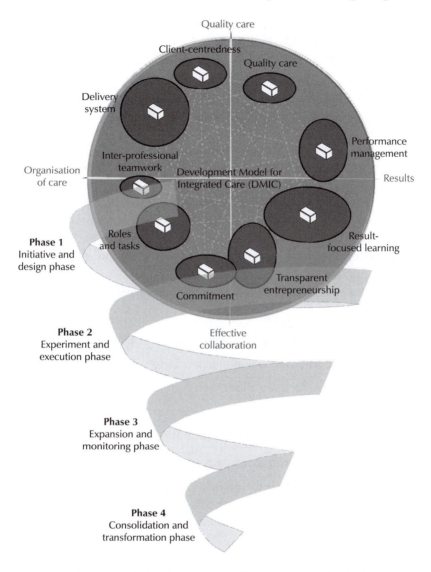

Figure 6.1: The Development Model for Integrated Care (DMIC)

Partnership Assessment Tool (PAT)

The PAT was developed by the Nuffield Institute at the University of Leeds to provide a simple, quick and cost-effective way of assessing the effectiveness of partnership working (Hardy, Hudson and Waddington 2003). It enables a rapid appraisal (a quick 'health check') that graphically identifies problem areas. This allows partners to focus remedial action and resources commensurate with the seriousness and urgency of the problems. Using the PAT therefore avoids exhaustive, lengthy and costly investigations of partnership working in general. For those just setting up partnerships, it provides a checklist of what to ensure and what to avoid. It has been designed explicitly as a developmental tool rather than as a means for centrally assessing local partnership performance.

The tool can be used to assess partnership working at different levels, for example with those at the highest level (elected member or board level), at senior/middle management level and amongst frontline staff (those who need to make the partnership work in practice). Repeating the exercise at different levels within the partnership provides the opportunity to compare and contrast views and to target remedial action where it is most needed. Also, repeating the exercise over time allows partnerships to chart their progress in addressing problems and achieving their goals.

The principles on which it is based are generic. It is therefore applicable in a wide range of contexts. These principles are as follows:

- Principle 1: Recognise and accept the need for partnership

- Principle 2: Develop clarity and realism of purpose

- Principle 3: Ensure commitment and ownership

- Principle 4: Develop and maintain trust

- Principle 5: Create clear and robust partnership arrangements

- Principle 6: Monitor, measure and learn.

It is designed to be used in four stages:

- 1st stage: Agreeing the purpose of the tool. Is the process to be mainly developmental, more of a routine audit, or part of a more extensive remedial programme?

- 2nd stage: Partners will need to become familiar with the material. Experience suggests that independent, though not necessarily external, facilitation is helpful in managing the process and encouraging openness in partners. Partners read the material and carry out the exercise individually if they prefer or if it is difficult to bring partners together. In completing the assessment exercise each partner will complete the six rapid assessment profile sheets, indicating their responses to a set of statements grouped under each of the six partnership principles.

- 3rd stage: Analysis of these responses and the generation of a partnership profile.

- 4th stage: Results of the analysis can then be shared and discussed with partners in a workshop. This gives partners the chance to look in more detail at their assessments and their particular judgements about individual statements.

At this stage, action planning can be undertaken to identify and agree any remedial action.

How can you learn from and share your findings?

At the beginning of this chapter we highlighted the common experience of evaluative review processes not being embedded within an initiative. It is similarly common that when a review is complete, the results are not shared in a timely manner or actively used to promote learning and improvement. The contributory factors are similar – a pressure on getting on with the day job meaning that there is never time to complete the report or to hold the event, the pace of development leading to the findings being seen to reflect what was the case rather than current practice, and a lack of confidence in how best to enthuse others about what has been discovered. Once again, there is no one way to do this. It is important to start with the overall aims of the evaluative review and its target stakeholders and audiences, and to embed learning and dissemination from the beginning of the process (see Case example 6.7). Being clear with participants as to how you will share the findings, and giving them at least access to these, is also good ethical practice.

Interim and final reports are often the main expected outputs from an evaluative review. The Standards for QUality Improvement Reporting Excellence (SQUIRE 2.) (Ogrinc *et al.* 2015) sets out the key content that should be covered within such reports:

- *Why did you start?* The initial problem or issue, what was previously known, the rationale behind the approach, and the aims of the project and report.

- *What did you do?* Important contextual elements, sufficient detail of the initiative to enable others to understand what was planned, the study design and methods, how data was analysed, and the response to ethical issues.

- *What did you find?* The evolution of the initiative over time, interaction between the initiative and the context, association between impact and interventions, and any unintended consequences.

- *What does it mean?* A summary of key findings, whether the initial assumptions and expectations were realised, what lay behind any differences, limitations to the evaluative review, how useful the findings were, and potential for adoption elsewhere.

As well as the content, the tone and style of the reports are important. Many integrated care initiative leaders will be familiar with writing organisational reports that deploy formal language and can be somewhat dry. Whilst this may be appropriate for the evaluative review report, it may also be possible to write in a more engaging manner. If the results are to be shared more widely, it is important to think about the reading ability and communication needs of the expected audience – it is also worth being realistic about how long you are likely to hold someone's interest for (even if you find the results fascinating)! Accessible summaries are usually a must, therefore, and *infographics* can be an attractive way of presenting the key facts. Formats other than written reports are also worth considering, with short videos providing an overview of the main learning being helpful accompaniments on websites. Promoting through social media such as Twitter is an easy and free way to inform and engage people.

To support local learning it can be helpful to have a framework in mind for how this could be undertaken. Two tried and tested frameworks are those of 'action research' and the 'Plan, Do, Study, Act' (PDSA) cycle. These have been developed through different routes – action research from the field of organisational development and change, and PDSA through operational management and improvement. They both, though, depict a circular process in which the need for change is explored, the thinking behind the change is mapped, data is gathered to understand what has actually happened, and the intervention or approach is adapted accordingly. This cycle is then repeated in relation to the adapted intervention (see Figure 6.2). Action research also emphasises the importance of engaging stakeholders in the analysis and decision-making processes rather than 'designated experts' undertaking these tasks in isolation. As reflected in Case example 6.7, such learning cycles can operate at different levels simultaneously, with services undertaking these with 'meso' and 'micro' initiatives, and the programme as a whole distilling these at a macro level for the organisation or partnership.

The PDSA cycle is a four-stage process-improvement model used to rapidly trial planned changes to practice, incorporate the lessons learned from the trial into the change process, and integrate continuous improvement into the new service.

Stages in the PDSA Cycle

1. *Planning:* This initial stage requires a thorough diagnostic evaluation of the problems/issues that need to be addressed by the change – firstly to identify their probable causes and secondly to design possible solutions.

2. *Doing:* A small-scale (pilot) project is undertaken as a limited implementation of the proposed change(s). Data is collected and observations made to identify the impact of the change and any unintended consequences.

3. *Studying:* Results of the pilot are compared with expectations to identify unintended consequences and shortfalls in improvements.

4. *Acting:* Improvements to the proposed intervention are made, incorporating lessons learned from the pilot phase. The changes may be tested again in another pilot, or the decision taken to proceed to full implementation. Ongoing quality improvement activity (continuous cycles) may also be adopted.

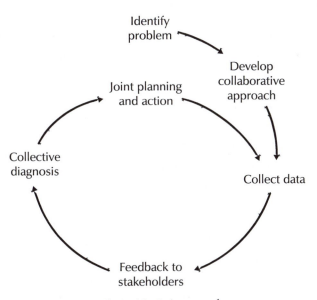

Figure 6.2: Action research

Case example 6.7: Evaluation of the Achieving Clinical Excellence (ACE) pioneer programme

The ACE programme was designed by the clinical commissioning group (CCG) to encourage 'pioneer' groups of GPs to develop enhanced primary care services. Its goals were to improve patient experience through providing locally based diagnostic and treatment services, to improve the health of patients with multiple conditions, and to achieve cost savings through diverting activity from acute to primary care. A dual evaluation and review were completed to understand if the programme was achieving these objectives, and to gather learning for the further roll-out of the approach and any successful pilot initiatives that were developed by practice. It was also hoped that the external evaluators would act as 'critical friends' to the process, and use emerging findings to help participants reflect on progress, barriers and opportunities.

An external team based within a university undertook the evaluation element. The university was responsible for gathering the experiences of the pioneer groups. They did this through interviewing the leads of the individual pioneers and the key leads within the CCG at three, six and nine months, and observing monthly learning sets. Feedback was provided by the university on a periodic basis on the key issues that had arisen in order that the pioneers and commissioners could respond to these. The CCG completed the review element. They identified and analysed datasets that could be used to assess changes in relevant outcomes and activies. They also undertook a performance appraisal of each pioneer at the end of the programme. The evaluation and review findings were collated in a final report to the board of the commissioning organisation, with clear implications for future such improvement initiatives. Following further interviews six months post-programme, they will be used to produce a public report and academic article.

What does this case example tell us?

» This evaluation demonstrates the action research cycle in practice, with regular gathering, analysis and sharing of data to inform further implementation.

» The cycle was used by the individual pioneers in relation to their local initiatives and by the CCG in relation to the whole programme.

» It highlights how the evaluation and review elements can be combined with different organisations undertaking the elements that best reflect their role and skills.

Chapter 7

Working with Service Users and Carers

This chapter focuses on the kind of involvement where the focus is more about improving people's lives, by having more say over the services they use and more control over their lives in general and, by so doing, bringing about broader social and political change – also known as the 'democratic' approach. This is the second reason why we should engage and involve people in health and social care, and is different to the first reason – the 'consumerist' approach, covered earlier in Chapter 3.

In this chapter we consider what integrated services might look like if the service user really is at the heart of services, and what you might need to think about, and do, in order to achieve this. We also explore some fundamental principles that should underpin whatever it is that you do.

In this chapter we cover the following:

- What is the difference between self-efficacy, personal activation and advocacy?

- How can we support people to be 'self-caring' and 'self-managing'?

- What contribution can peer support networks make to integrated care?

- Is it possible to put people at the centre of decisions about their care?

- How can we design services in true partnership with service users?

What is the difference between self-efficacy, personal activation and advocacy?

Self-efficacy

Self-efficacy (Bandura 1995) is used to describe the confidence people have that they can successfully carry out specific actions or tasks to achieve a desired goal. If you have a strong sense of self-efficacy, you may view challenging problems with relish, and are also likely to develop a much deeper interest in, and commitment to, the activities that you undertake. You are more likely to recover quickly from setbacks and disappointments. However, if you have a weak sense of self-efficacy, you may find yourself avoiding challenging tasks because you believe that difficult tasks and situations are beyond your capabilities. You focus on your personal failings and negative outcomes, and quickly lose confidence in your personal abilities.

Self-efficacy can impact on everything from psychological state to behaviour to motivation – all of which will have a direct impact on how individuals think and feel about their health and wellbeing and how involved they might wish to be in activities concerning their own health and wellbeing. This could include day-to-day concerns about healthy eating and taking regular exercise, to setting specific health goals and planning personal care packages.

Activation

There are close links between self-efficacy and activation – the belief in oneself and the carrying out of specific actions. The concept of activation comes from Judith Hibbard *et al.*'s (2004) work on patient activation and the development of a tool by which people's level of activation can be measured. The first step in someone being 'activated' is the recognition that they have an important role to play in their own health and wellbeing, whilst the next stage is having the confidence and knowledge necessary to take whatever action is appropriate. The third stage is actually taking action to maintain and improve one's health and wellbeing, whilst the final stage is staying the course, even under stress. Research suggests that more highly activated patients engage in healthier behaviour and experience better health, so this is an important concept to be aware of and to take into consideration when developing interventions to help people take more control over their health and wellbeing.

Activation can be increased through a range of tailored interventions such as peer support and coaching that recognises where people 'are at', and works with them on their terms, rather than imposing unrealistic goals or targets (see Case example 7.1). It is only when the level of a person's activation is understood that health messages can be targeted, consistent and effective. For example, if an overweight, diabetic smoker who does not feel that they have an active role to play in their health and who is disposed to be a passive recipient of healthcare (level 1 activation) attends their GP for a consultation for backache and is told to lose weight, cut out sugary foods, take more exercise and stop smoking, they are likely to be overwhelmed by the scale of what they must do, and consequently do nothing.

This becomes an even more important concept when service users are in receipt of a range of services potentially from a number of different organisations, and are therefore trying to find a way through a confusing landscape of services, organisations and people.

Case example 7.1: Southend Clinical Commissioning Group (CCG) – Patient Activation Measures (PAM) pilot

Long-term conditions are a particular concern in Southend-on-Sea, as it has an older population than the England average, and higher levels of deprivation than the country as a whole. It also has a higher number of people with three or more long-term conditions (12.9%, compared to the national average of 10.5%).

A pilot PAM and Social Prescribing intervention was commissioned in seven Southend GP practices as part of the town's integrated health and social care pioneer project and its health and wellbeing strategy. The aim of the programme is to empower people with long-term conditions to address negative lifestyle or behavioural risk factors to improve their health and wellbeing, and to reduce the unnecessary use of health and social care resources.

With help from Self Management UK, patient invitation letters and instructions to complete the PAM questionnaire have been sent to over 8000 patients with long-term conditions.

What does this case example tell us?
Identifying people's activation levels will help inform the CCG of the subsequent interventions that are most likely to support them with self-management of their conditions. This should enable the CCG to prioritise interventions and get best value for patients and service users.

Advocacy

Advocacy provides people with the support they need to help them express their views and wishes. Sometimes people find it difficult for a whole range of reasons to express themselves and to have their voices heard. Generally speaking, an advocate will listen to people's views and concerns, give information and help signpost people to different services or support, help them consider different options and make choices, and liaise between service users and services. An advocate can accompany service users to meetings or appointments and may speak on their behalf.

It is also important to recognise what advocacy is not – it is not about giving someone their personal opinion about what they should or shouldn't do. It is not about solving people's problems or making decisions on their behalf.

In an integrated care setting, an advocate can help someone in exactly the same way, but their involvement might be particularly beneficial in supporting someone to understand this different kind of approach, where one team or organisation might be delivering care and services previously delivered by several different people or organisations.

There are various different types of advocacy. People can choose to be their own advocate (self-advocacy), they can ask a friend, family member or carer to act on their behalf, or they can access a professional advocacy service. There is also peer advocacy, where people who have experience of problems can support others with the same problems, such as the Older People's Advocacy Alliance (OPAAL) programme for older people with cancer.

In some circumstances people might have a legal right to an advocate, such as an independent mental health advocate (IMHA), which is called statutory advocacy. And some charities or organisations provide advocacy for specific issues; for example, Shelter offers advocacy for people with housing problems, whilst Rethink Mental Illness provides mental health advocacy services in the community, secure hospitals and secure units.

As a practitioner, it is useful to know what advocacy services are available. There are a number of organisations that can provide such support, and these are listed at the end of this book. It is also useful to remember that you may well be working with people who have advocates, and that their involvement may need to be factored into the planning of any involvement activity.

How can we support people to be 'self-caring' and 'self-managing'?

The increasing rates of chronic disease in the population, its impact on people's daily lives and the need to contain costs means that people are being actively encouraged to take more responsibility and control over their own health and wellbeing, and to become more involved in looking after themselves and keeping well.

Self-care and self-management are often used interchangeably, but it might be helpful to think of them as two distinct concepts. Self-care refers to the activities that enable people to deal with the impact on their daily lives of having a long-term condition, such as dealing with any emotional consequences, adhering to treatment regimes and maintaining activities that are important to them, such as work, socialising and being with and looking after family. It can also include people's ability to undertake activities of daily living such as washing, dressing, shopping and preparing meals. The Department of Health's definition of self-care is as follows: 'The actions people take for themselves, their children and their families to stay fit and maintain good physical and mental health; meet social and psychological needs; prevent illness or accidents; care for minor ailments and long term conditions; and maintain health and wellbeing after an acute illness or discharge from hospital' (DH 2005, p.1).

Meanwhile, self-management has been defined as 'the individual's ability to manage the symptoms, treatment, physical and psychosocial consequences and lifestyle changes inherent in living with a chronic condition' (Barlow *et al.* 2002, p.178). This might mean coping with the isolation and depression that often occurs alongside ill health, managing dietary restrictions or medication, or being aware of changes in how they are feeling in case they are beginning to experience some escalation in their condition.

People could be considered to be taking part in self-management-type activities in a range of ways, and the list below, shown in Figure 7.1, gives some examples of these, starting with the more medicalised types of activities, progressing through to the more social.

If you are providing an integrated service, it is likely that your service users are involved in a number of these activities, perhaps to varying degrees of efficacy, depending on their activation, and a coordinated approach to supporting people to undertake these activities will be important. Just keeping a record of the activities they might be engaged in so that everyone involved in their care is aware of them can prove challenging, but worthwhile.

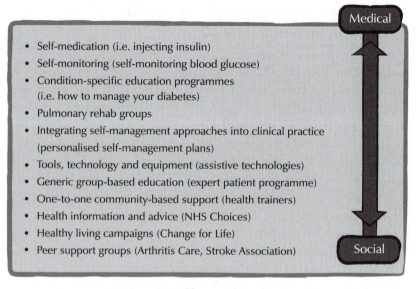

Figure 7.1: Self-management spectrum

The term 'expert patient' or 'expert service user' is often used for people who have had their condition for some length of time, and who have developed a reputation for being engaged in their condition. They are recognised by care professionals as having some legitimacy as spokespeople for their condition. However, the term can be contentious, as it is assumed that in order to be an 'expert', a body of knowledge is required. The kind of knowledge required is often judged through the lens of a clinical professional, rather than recognising that it is the experience of living with the condition that defines 'expertise'. The term 'expert by experience' is therefore also used, and has gained more currency in recent years.

Whatever term you use, it is important when working with people in these circumstances to understand their individual situation and point of view, in order to identify solutions that are determined by them as leading to good outcomes, and not solutions that are determined as being the same for everyone with the same condition. For example, evidence shows that when it comes to medicine compliance, an individual's personal beliefs, priorities and attitudes to risk determine compliance, not whether someone is an 'expert' service user.

It is also worth reminding ourselves that people living with a long-term condition spend the vast majority of their time coping with their condition on their own, or with the support of family and carers, rather than with the intervention of health and social care professionals. The contribution of your service to someone's care in this sense may be important, but it is very small. For example, there are a minimum 672 hours in a month. Let's assume someone with a chronic condition might, in an average month, attend one clinical appointment of some description for 30 minutes, and they attend some sort of support-type group for two hours a fortnight. Let's also assume that they have a visit from a health or social care professional for 30 minutes every week – all of this equates to just 6.5 hours a month, a fraction less than 1 per cent of the total time in the month. Even if they have home help for two hours a day, that's still less than 10 per cent of the time.

It's vitally important therefore to support people to develop their ability to self-care and self-manage, as they are the most constant resource available to them. This involves a number of elements, not least the provision of accurate and up-to-date information for service users about their condition and the services available to them. One of the ways in which this might be achieved is by providing people with access to their full medical records, as in the example from the US presented in Case example 7.2.

Case example 7.2: Access to records in the US

This initiative gives five million US citizens access to their full medical records online. Patients are advised when their primary care doctor has added notes to their records, and they receive reminders to review them. Of the participating population, 82 per cent of patients had accessed at least one of their notes, and this included older people, those with poorer health status and those with lower educational attainment. Less than 8 per cent said that reading their notes made them feel worried or confused. Three-quarters of people reported taking better care of themselves and feeling more in control of their care, better prepared for clinical appointments and better able to understand how to take their medications.

After a year of the pilot, 99 per cent of patients wanted to continue to see their notes online.

What does this case example tell us?

» Access to medical records can enable people to become more engaged with their healthcare.

» Access to medical records can activate people to take more health-promoting behaviour.

» Access to medical records can help to develop a different, more productive relationship between the service user and health or social care practitioner.

» Early findings suggest that full access to medical records could become a core element of coordinated care systems.

What contribution can peer support networks make to integrated care?

Social participation and supportive social networks are increasingly recognised as important for illness management, especially long-term conditions (Vassilev et al. 2014). There is evidence that, in general, the likelihood of survival for those with a long-term condition is higher in people with strong social relationships. Social networks are systems of support that have a range of functions – network members exert positive influences on self-management by giving indirect help with medication, supporting a healthy diet and exercise, playing an active role during doctors' visits, providing transport, sharing illness-related information, talking about shared situations, offering understanding, and motivating older adults to follow a prescribed regimen.

Research suggests that people who are meaningfully engaged in things beyond family and friends have greater access to health-relevant support, and are more accessible to interventions and more able to adapt to new health practices (Vassilev et al. 2013). It also shows that greater social involvement is significantly related to better self-management ability, better physical health and greater emotional wellbeing (Reeves et al. 2014).

Social networks are of particular relevance for self-care support or management as it moves the focus away from an individual's self-management to a broader consideration of all the resources available to help someone. It may be useful to take this into account when considering how to make the best use of resources, although research suggests that whilst peer support helps people cope practically and emotionally with their condition, it does not necessarily impact on health needs per se. Self-management support from within the community has, however, been shown to be effective for groups who may otherwise be difficult to reach, and those who are culturally or linguistically diverse (see Figure 7.2).

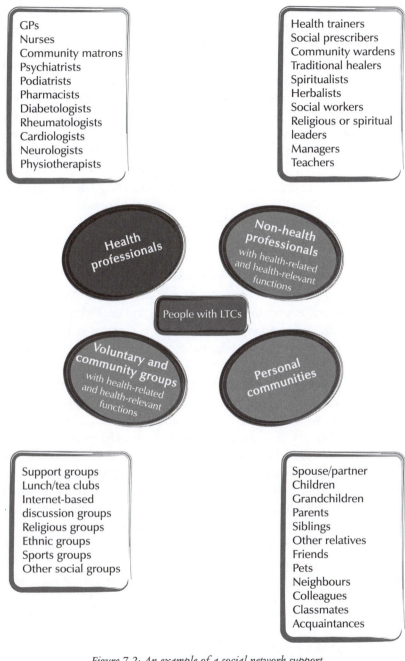

GPs
Nurses
Community matrons
Psychiatrists
Podiatrists
Pharmacists
Diabetologists
Rheumatologists
Cardiologists
Neurologists
Physiotherapists

Health trainers
Social prescribers
Community wardens
Traditional healers
Spiritualists
Herbalists
Social workers
Religious or spiritual
leaders
Managers
Teachers

Health professionals

Non-health professionals with health-related and health-relevant functions

People with LTCs

Voluntary and community groups with health-related and health-relevant functions

Personal communities

Support groups
Lunch/tea clubs
Internet-based
discussion groups
Religious groups
Ethnic groups
Sports groups
Other social groups

Spouse/partner
Children
Grandchildren
Parents
Siblings
Other relatives
Friends
Pets
Neighbours
Colleagues
Classmates
Acquaintances

*Figure 7.2: An example of a social network support
system for people with long-term conditions*
Source: Rogers *et al.* (2014)

Peer support can be provided as part of a group programme facilitated by health professionals and/or through professionally organised or self-help support groups. An evaluation of the UK-based Expert Patients Programme showed improvements in participants' self-efficacy and energy and better psychological wellbeing, although no significant difference in the use of health services (Kennedy *et al.* 2007), whilst a peer support intervention for diabetic patients (Piette *et al.* 2013) improved glycaemic control largely due to them being more likely to inject insulin when needed. This latter intervention had its greatest benefits amongst patients with low support or poorer health literacy. There are examples and case studies of condition-specific groups such as stroke support clubs enhancing self-management by creating a safe and supportive environment that encourages people to try new things for themselves without fear of ridicule, and that motivate people to recover as far as they can, as they test their progress out against their fellow participants.

It is also reported that 'trusted environments' afforded by online communities and peer support groups can help men in particular to overcome cultural expectations of masculinity and enable them to 'open up' emotionally. Peer support can offer men a sense of belonging and community, and can help them adjust and come to terms with their health problems (Galdas *et al.* 2014).

The emergence of online social networks, for example #DOC on Twitter for people with diabetes, can also be particularly helpful to individuals with lower patient activation (Magnezi, Bergman and Grosberg 2014). For practitioners working with older people to take a more active role in self-care and self-management, it is useful to know that research supports attention being paid to identify the positive and negative influences from service users' social networks, and the inclusion of positively influential social network members in the healthcare encounter in order to increase adherence to a management regimen.

So, in summary, greater social involvement and social peer support can lead to better self-management ability, better physical health and greater emotional wellbeing, and practitioners should consider how involvement in these networks can be both encouraged and supported.

Is it possible to put people at the centre of decisions about their care?

The concept of personalised care and support planning has now been part of the rhetoric about how things are done within health and social care for many years, but in reality, its implementation in a genuine and meaningful way remains patchy.

The concept of a person-centred approach to care planning is rooted in the concepts of rights, independence and choice. Put simply, person-centred care planning means that planning starts with the individual and what their needs and preferences are, and not with the services and what is available. The concept is not limited to health and social care services, but includes housing, education, employment and leisure. Delivering this approach requires real organisational cultural change and changes in practice, replacing a culture of paternalism with personally tailored services, where people have choice, control and power over the services they receive. Evidence also shows that personalised care and support planning can lead to the most appropriate use of limited healthcare resources.

Official government guidance provides a useful framework for service leads and commissioners, but the essence of this is the ability to listen to service users and their carers to find out what is important to them and to think creatively about responding to these needs and preferences, without being constrained by structural concepts of what 'the service' is that is being provided. In an integrated care context, person-centred planning will draw on the creativity and contribution of a range of people, as the service user's holistic needs are considered, and not just their health or social care needs.

The House of Care approach (see Figure 7.3) is used as a framework to help practitioners and commissioners think about what needs to be in place to support the changes that need to happen culturally and in practice to deliver person-centred planning and personalised care. It relies on four key interdependent components, all of which, it is suggested, must be present for person-centred coordinated care to be realised. These four components are:

- *Commissioning:* Seen as a service improvement process and not simply a procurement process.

- *Engaged, informed individuals and carers:* Enabling individuals to self-manage and know how to access the services they need when and where they need them.

- *Organisational and clinical processes:* Structured around the needs of patients and carers using the best evidence available, co-designed with service users where possible.

- *Health and care professionals working in partnership:* Listening, supporting and collaborating for continuity of care.

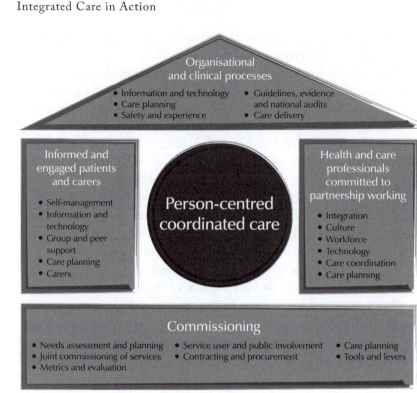

Figure 7.3: House of Care

In order to achieve this, the integrated care team will need to have discussions with service users about what is important to them, what goals they want to work towards, what they can do to live well and stay well, what they can do for themselves and what they need support with, and finally, preparing for the future (see Case examples 7.3 and 7.4). A range of professionals, or an advocate or a volunteer, may initiate these conversations, but they do need to be recorded so that they can be shared with care-givers and other relevant parties (with the service user's consent), for their benefit. The conversations could be planned or may be impromptu, and it is therefore important to consider managing these kinds of conversations as a generic skill for all members of an integrated care team to develop, rather than something that only one or two people in the team can do.

Person-centred planning is another approach that can help service users to think through what is important to them and then work with care teams and other professionals to make these happen in practice (Bowers *et al.* 2007). There are a number of different frameworks that can be used to structure the planning process, but all of them have at their heart the same principles of stating what is important to the person, giving time and support for communication, and drawing together not only professionals and practitioners, but also the people who are important in their lives. Person-centred plans can be successfully combined with personal budgets, where the service user is notified of the funding available to them and is able to direct how this is spent to meet their hopes and needs. The funding can be paid direct to the service user or an identified circle of support of people that they trust, or can be held by the lead provider in the form of an individual service fund (Sanderson and Miller 2014).

Case example 7.3: Care planning for people with long-term care needs – Holmside Medical Group

Holmside is a 9000-person, inner-city practice in Newcastle. It started to introduce care and support planning for their long-term care patients in 2012, by working with the Year of Care Partnership.[1] The whole practice team worked to reorganise systems and develop staff to introduce an approach that focuses on what matters to each person in their daily lives, what they would like to achieve, and what support is needed, all brought together in a single process and plan.

These changes required staff to take on new roles. For example, administrative staff were trained to be able to help people navigate the care system, healthcare assistants play a key role in explaining the care planning process and roles to patients, as well as signposting people to supportive community activities, whilst the nursing team use their consultation skills to identify what is important to each person, supporting them to find solutions and practical actions. As a result of introducing this approach, the practice has found that people are more involved in the care planning process as well as with their own health.

What does this case example tell us?

» Introducing a more personalised care planning process will require some fundamental changes within an organisation.

» Commitment to make a difference must be present at all levels – everyone has a role to play.

» Such an approach can pay significant dividends in terms of people's engagement with their own health.

---

1   The Year of Care Partnership is a programme to develop the evidence base for a capitated budget approach for people with long-term conditions. See www.yearofcare.co.uk

Case example 7.4: Care planning for vulnerable people – Living Well Programme, Cornwall

In Cornwall they are exploring new ways to integrate services in order to improve the quality of life for the most vulnerable. A partnership has been created between the voluntary and community sector, the local authority and health commissioners and providers, and its focus is on creating a service that goes beyond health and social care, to include emotional wellbeing, financial stability, and social connectivity and purpose for people.

Each person will receive a different, tailored service – underpinned by the principles of listening to individual stories and ensuring people get the health and social care they need in a way that puts their needs before that of the organisation. The programme presents challenges to all those involved in delivering services such as information sharing, attitudes to risk and the pace of change, but positive changes have already been developed. For example, the local voluntary and community sector is now able, with appropriate consent, to access NHS records, NHS numbers are in use in social care systems, and partners are all taking a coordinated approach to how they ask service users for their consent for information to be shared.

What does this case example tell us?

» In order to deliver a truly integrated person-centred approach, all organisations involved have to make changes to the way they operate. This might include some quite fundamental changes to behaviours and attitudes as well as processes and protocols.

» This requires a coordinated approach at the system-wide level, and will require vision and leadership.

» Maintaining such relationships requires energy and commitment, but harnessing the voice of the service user as a driver and motivator for sustained change can be powerful.

How can we design services in true partnership with service users?

Co-production is another one of those terms that is quite difficult to define. It is not a new concept, and stems from recognition that public services are joint endeavours of government and citizens, and that the production and consumption of such services are inseparable.

It often means different things to different people, but for the purposes of this book, we define it as the process by which service users and those commissioning or providing services come together as equal partners to develop mutually agreed solutions to the inherent problems that exist in the delivery of public services. There is a difference between co-production and involvement in terms of degree, so whilst co-production is an involvement activity, not all involvement activities could be said to be co-produced. Co-production might include co-design, including the planning of services, co-decision-making in terms of the allocation of resources, co-delivery of services and co-evaluation of services.

However co-production is applied in practice, there are a number of principles that should underpin such activities, as follows. Service users are seen as active asset-holders rather than passive consumers; co-production promotes collaborative rather than paternalistic relationships between staff and service users, so that power is shared; the focus is on the delivery of outcomes rather than services; and co-production is based on the concept of reciprocity (an equal exchange of input and outcomes) and mutuality (people working together to achieve their shared interests). There is also an implicit understanding that service users are included in any activity or project that affects them from the very start to the end.

Co-production is not without controversy, however, as some have suggested that it is unfair to expect people to put their time, energy and effort into co-production, particularly if they are vulnerable or disadvantaged, whilst others have suggested that, in practice, real power sharing is unlikely, so that co-production efforts can rarely be truly equal.

Co-production may be substitutive in that it focuses on replacing local government inputs by inputs from service users or communities, or additive in that it adds more service user or community inputs to professional inputs or it introduces professional support where it has not been present previously, such as self-help groups. There is also a debate as to whether co-production is relational or transactional, whereby the former requires the active involvement and decision-making of service users in collaboration with others, and the latter requires collaborative behaviours rather than personal interactions between service users and public sector staff (see Table 7.1).

Table 7.1: Different resource implications for different types of co-production

Types of co-production		Resources brought by professionals and users/communities	
		Additive	Substitutive
Nature of interaction	**Relational**	Professionals and users doing joint assessment of user needs and care plans	Peer support networks of expert patients
	Transactional	Participatory budgeting done online ('e-PB') with citizens submitting proposals for community projects/public services	Doing initial illness diagnosis from professionally supported website

Source: Löffler (2010)

There is also a distinction made in the literature between personal co-production and community co-production. Personal co-production is closely linked to the concept of personal budgets and the ability of individuals to self-determine the services they need and what form these take, whereas community co-production is seen as being linked to volunteering, albeit people taking part in community co-production events might not recognise their actions as volunteering, even though they are giving their time for free.

Personal co-production results in personal as well as community value, whereas community co-production results in some specific instrumental outcomes, such as a consensus on how priorities should be determined, or resources allocated, but can also result in more productive relationships between people and service deliverers, and the development of trust, understanding and empathy.

There are few evaluations on co-production approaches in the literature, and there is much that is not known, such as the appetite of the general population to take part in such activities and, of those that do take part, what their motivations and expectations are. However, research suggests that people do tend to believe that services are better for the engagement of citizens (see Case example 7.5). Little is also known about the experiences of staff that participate in such activities.

For practitioners thinking about introducing co-production into their service area, or considering how to make existing co-production activities more sustainable or meaningful, there are a number of questions to ask, as follows:

- What skills do service users and citizens need in order to be able to co-produce outcomes effectively?

- What incentives can be used to encourage co-productive participation or behaviours?

- How do staff need to be supported in their potential roles as co-production facilitators?

- What information needs to be exchanged between professionals and service users in order to make co-production activities meaningful and productive?

- What other resources are required to support these activities?

- What resources will these activities bring into the organisation?

- What will be the 'cost' to individuals taking part in co-production activities, and can these costs be justified?

- How can the value of co-production outcomes be assessed?

Case example 7.5: North West London (NWL) integrated care programme – impact of lay partners

NWL have been integrating physical, mental and social care provision for elderly and diabetic patients for some time. There was already a patients, carers and users group, but NWL had ambitions to increase the scope and scale of engagement and involvement by co-designing the new system from the start, with patients/users/carers and other citizens.

An advisory group of 20 lay partners was recruited from amongst patients, carers and users who already had some experience of being involved in previous activities, and who felt able to undertake the commitment of more regular involvement. Some members came from the existing group whilst others were nominated via clinical commissioning groups (CCGs), Healthwatch, adult social services, primary care patient participation groups and patient charities. A full day of training for potential lay partners by a patient-led organisation was provided, and expenses incurred were remunerated.

All of the design workstreams and the overarching programme board for the redesign programme have had 1–3 lay partners as full members from the first meeting. On average, lay partners attend eight hours of meetings per month, as well as reading and commenting on discussion papers. Lay partners have developed a 'co-production touchstone', setting out principles and best practice for their involvement, and a number of lay partners co-chair their workstream. Their major impact is reported as keeping the focus of the programme on designing patient-centred, accessible, proactive and high-quality care.

What does this case example tell us?

» NWL was committed to involving service users, carers and citizens from the outset.

» Training was organised to enable people to contribute, and their costs of taking part were reimbursed.

» The commitment from lay partners is substantial, and this was flagged up at the recruitment stage to enable people to make their own decisions about taking part.

» The co-production touchstone suggests a genuine attempt to build trust and mutual respect.

» The co-chair arrangement suggests a genuine attempt to power share.

Experience-based design (EBD) is a specific form of co-production whereby service users and staff are brought together to tell and hear each other's stories, to identify 'touchpoints', and to redesign pathways and processes. It takes the concept of good design principles that bring together performance (function – is it fit for purpose, and does it do what it says it will do?), safety (is it safe and reliable?) and aesthetics (usability – how does it feel?), and applies them to health and care services (Bate and Robert 2006). So EBD is not just about the process and things such as waiting times to access services and duplicated assessments and tests, etc., but about feelings such as how people are communicated with and how they are made to feel in relation to certain processes or interactions with services. In EBD, the user experience is the starting point for authenticity. In the design of events, service users, carers and staff are first kept separate to narrate their experiences, and then they are brought together to share these narratives before agreeing what they will work together on changing.

For practitioners interested in introducing this kind of activity, it is important to recognise that capturing people's stories takes time, and it also takes understanding and skilled facilitation. This is particularly the case when experiences are subsequently shared between service users and staff. This sort of exercise might also take longer than anticipated, as it should be allowed to evolve rather than having time constraints applied – this can be particularly problematic if professionals feel they do not have permission to be absent from the frontline for 'as long as it takes'. It can also cost more than traditional ways of producing information.

Asset–based approaches to health and wellbeing and community development

Asset-based approaches are concerned with facilitating people and communities to come together to achieve positive change and to gain more control over their lives and circumstances, including the promotion of good health, by consciously and purposively using their own knowledge, skills and lived experience of the issues they encounter. This approach is the opposite to that of considering the deficits of individuals and communities and how they can be 'fixed' or treated. Assets could include the practical skills, capacity, knowledge and interests of local residents; their networks and connections; the presence of local community and voluntary associations; and the resources of public, private and third sector organisations that are available to support a community.

An asset-based approach emphasises the need to redress the balance between meeting needs and making people dependent and disempowered, so rather than people being seen just as consumers of health and care, they are also seen as co-producers. It is about nurturing the strengths and resources of people and communities, and promoting capacity, connectedness and social capital – enhancing the quality and longevity of life by focusing on those resources that promote the self-esteem and coping abilities of individuals and communities. Asset-based approaches will require changes in individual and organisational attitudes, values and practice, and are not simple change programmes to introduce.

Adopting an asset-based approach should be community-led, though in practice this is rarely the case, and the initiative is usually introduced and 'managed' by a government agency or its proxy. Asset-based approaches are by their very nature long-term, open-ended commitments, and will have varied, less easily defined, less easily measured and sometimes unpredictable outcomes, which are likely to take time to emerge. The exact approach needs to be context-specific and will require careful consideration and negotiation between individuals, communities and organisations. There is no 'one size fits all' approach, as it should be a bottom-up way of working that harnesses whatever local assets exist.

Some commentators are critical of these approaches, and suggest that they are a convenient excuse by which the government or statutory organisation can withdraw or limit services and leave people and communities often with complex needs to fend for themselves. Proponents are clear, though, that asset-based approaches are not about substitution or replacement of traditional health and care interventions, but should be complementary and embedded alongside such interventions. They are also clear that they are not a 'no cost' or money saving option.

It is certainly difficult to measure the impact of such approaches, as there is currently little evidence from large-scale research studies of their effectiveness. It is also difficult in this kind of approach to clearly demonstrate attribution. However, there is quite a library of case studies that is being built up and which demonstrate an impact in many different ways, whether by developing specific practical or life skills, or helping people into further training or employment.

To conclude this chapter, it may be useful to reflect on the point made in the section on self-care and self-management earlier. The interaction people have with statutory services represents a very small proportion of their lives. You cannot be all things to all people, all of the time. It is therefore useful to know about the range of possibilities that people can engage with, and to encourage, and where possible support, people to get involved.

Chapter 8

Working with Staff

For most integrated care initiatives one, or perhaps the, key resource that they will use to achieve better outcomes will be the staff working within the service. They are the main contact point that service users and their carers will have with the new arrangements, and are central to shaping people's experience of receiving support. Staff members will have unique insights regarding the current challenges faced by service users, carers and local communities, and through their experience and professional knowledge, to the potential solutions that could address any gaps or shortfalls. Taking a different perspective, as discussed in Chapter 5, they have the potential to disrupt or indeed effectively prevent new models of practice being introduced. Due to personal commitments and other connections with an area, many will work in the same locality for many years, meaning that they can outlast changes in policy or service reconfigurations, and so can provide a remaining legacy of how to work with other professions and services. They are, furthermore, key stakeholders in their own right, whose welfare and future career hopes should also be considered and responded to.

Ensuring that staff members within an integrated care initiative are able to work positively within the service and so contribute their skills and knowledge is therefore a key consideration. This is clearly not dissimilar to other services within this sector, and so the leaders of the initiative should have experiences that they can draw on. There are, though, key added challenges to overseeing an integrated care initiative. It may incorporate a range of professions and functions that are unfamiliar and different to a manager's own background and experience. Dependent on their professional and employing organisation, there may be alternative sets of performance and development frameworks. They may not be based wholly on the initiative, but spend some of their time working in other services. Finally, evidence highlights that there are additional complexities regarding the workings of an integrated care initiative that must be considered and responded to.

We have previously explored the change process and how to positively engage staff through leadership and the management of change. In this chapter we focus on approaches that can be used to positively engage staff in the delivery of integrated care. The key questions considered are the following:

- What are the common difficulties in professions working together?

- What are the skills, knowledge and values required for inter-professional working?

- How can we understand organisational culture?

- How can we use supervision within an integrated care initiative?

- What contribution can training and development make?

- How can we develop good team working?

- Can communities of practice make a positive contribution?

What are the common difficulties in professions working together?

Healthcare services in particular are a rich tapestry of different professional groups – medics, nurses, therapists, psychologists and pharmacists, to name but a few. Furthermore, within these health professions there are often distinct specialisms related to different medical roles or conditions – surgeon, physician, geriatrician, psychiatrist and so on. Professions were created as a means to guarantee the quality of service that would be provided to a service user. This is generally achieved through requiring a minimum level of qualifications and experience, compliance with ongoing practice development and review, and registration with a recognised professional body. Therefore people who pursue such a career have to pass rigorous training lasting many years in which they become socialised into this profession's ways of thinking, communicating and values. They develop pride in their profession based on their inside knowledge of its particular skills and evidence base, and will have considerable loyalty to its status and role. Furthermore, professions can also be interpreted as a means to protect particular types of employment and therefore income to a discrete set of individuals. This could be seen to translate into professional groups wanting to maintain their own 'turf' from others in case this decreases their own ability to earn a good wage.

In social care and housing support there is a smaller range of formal professions, with social work and occupational therapy being the most common. There are, though, a number of frontline roles in these sectors and indeed in healthcare that may not meet the formal requirements to be a profession, but that must demonstrate a high level of competence and will have requirements regarding training and experience. Management is similarly not a distinct profession as such, although many such jobs now expect or at least prefer a relevant qualification. There are also 'true' professions within support functions such as accountants, lawyers and human resources (HR). All of this means that integrated care initiatives are likely to be a melting pot of professions and other groups who all believe in the importance of their role and the need for it to carry on in the future. Whilst in many ways this diversity is the strength of such a service, there are a number of issues related to 'professions' that commonly arise. Furthermore, it is also the case that bringing them together and especially co-locating them can lead to an intensification of these tensions. Key issues that can lead to such tensions are the following:

- *Skills and identity:* Professionals who are in a minority within an integrated care initiative can feel that they start to lose their particular skills and knowledge through being distant to others within their profession. This can make them feel that they are no longer as confident in being able to practise in such a role. They can also start to take on some of the ways of thinking and communicating of the professions that they are surrounded by, and even begin to express criticism of their own profession as a way of 'fitting in'.

- *Status and power:* Professional rivalries exist in most settings, as those from different groups attempt to get their ways of thinking recognised and seek to avoid domination by others. This is often a combination of believing in their perspective, not wanting their profession to be diluted, and the undoubted connection between status, salary and opportunity. Common rivalries are those between doctors and nurses, nurses and therapists, and social workers and just about everyone else! There is also a divide between the recognised professions and other roles.

- *Communication and understanding:* Professionals often find it difficult to translate what their perspective is to someone of another profession. This can be due to the different terminology and acronyms that are used, the specialist knowledge held by one but not by another, and the patterns of communication that are normally deployed. Perhaps more fundamentally, professions can have alternative ways of seeing the world and the needs of service users and their families, which means that they can be saying the same thing but mean something very different. It is striking how little professionals who have worked together for years actually know about each other.

- *Incentives and performance:* One of the by-products of the various professions developing in parallel is that they have been able to negotiate or been subjected to alternative systems of performance and (perhaps most importantly) pay. There are also similar issues connected with professions and roles employed by different organisations or sectors – so, for example, administration staff working for the NHS or local authority, or between those undertaking support roles within the statutory or voluntary sector. These are important in relation to the issues of status, and also because staff members who are seconded into an initiative may not feel that their frameworks are recognised and understood, which would put them at a disadvantage in terms of promotion and reward.

What are the skills, knowledge and values required for inter-professional working?

Being a professional, or indeed undertaking another role successfully, requires the individual concerned having a set of competences connected with their profession and/or role. Being competent is to demonstrate the necessary skills, knowledge and values required to practise to a good standard. For all professionals and practitioners this includes *complementary competences* that are central to their own professional role and that can be delivered alongside that of others. For example, nurses are able to administer medication, physiotherapists to recommend movements to strengthen physical recovery, and psychologists to provide therapeutic interventions. There are also a set of *common competences* that have to be demonstrated by most, if not all, professionals and practitioners, such as communicating with service users, treating people with respect, and making accurate and timely recordings (Barr 1998). An integrated care initiative entails another set of competences in working with those from other professional roles, sometimes termed *inter-professionality.*

Inter-professionality: The process by which professionals reflect on and develop ways of practicing that provides an integrated and cohesive answer to the needs of the client/family/population... [I]t involves continuous interaction and knowledge sharing between professionals, organized to solve or explore a variety of education and care issues all whilst seeking to optimize the patient's participation... Inter-professionality requires a paradigm shift, since inter-professional practice has unique characteristics in terms of values, codes of conduct, and ways of working. These characteristics must be elucidated. (D'Amour and Oandasan 2005, p.9)

There has been considerable work internationally to define these core inter-professional competences. The Inter-professional Education Collaborative in the US has developed a holistic model that incorporates the main findings from research and previous models. This has four domains, as shown in Table 8.1.

Table 8.1: Core inter-professional competences

Domain	Demonstrated through...
Work with individuals from other professions to maintain a climate of mutual respect and shared values	Acting with honesty and integrity, placing service users at the centre, embracing cultural diversity, respecting other professions and roles, demonstrating high ethical standards
Use the knowledge of one's own role and those of others to respond to the needs of service users and populations served	Clearly communicating one's roles and responsibilities, recognising own limitations, engaging other professions and roles as required, clarifying each other's responsibilities, engaging in professional and inter-professional development
Communicate with service users, carers, citizens and other professionals and roles in a responsive and responsible manner that supports a team approach	Choosing communication tools and techniques that facilitate team discussions and interactions, avoiding discipline-specific jargon where possible, expressing own knowledge and opinions clearly, actively listening and encouraging opinions from other team members, giving constructive feedback and responding to that received, using respectful language
Apply relationship-building values and principles of team dynamics to perform effectively as a team to provide a quality service	Developing consensus on ethical principles, engaging relevant others in shared problem-solving, applying leadership practices that support collaboration and team effectiveness, managing constructively disagreements that arise, sharing accountability for outcomes, reflecting on team and individual performance, using evidence within improvement processes

Source: Inter-professional Education Collaborative Expert Panel (2011)

How can we understand organisational culture?

It is hard to find an enquiry or review regarding poor care or abuse of vulnerable people that does not highlight that a poor or negative culture within the services and organisations has been a contributory factor. Equally, the need to ensure a positive culture is generally included within the recommendations of such investigations. The concept is also widely included in the vision of organisations and partnerships, and within national policy and practice guidance. Despite becoming such a central part of our thinking about how services work, there continues to be uncertainty about what culture actually is, and if we can change it for the better. For example, one issue of debate is the extent to which there is a common culture across organisations, with some commentators arguing that there are, in fact, a set of sub-cultures within different services and other groupings that can act as a support or resistor to the overall organisational direction. Others do not even see this level of solidity, and instead argue that there is not settled culture but, instead, numerous dynamic and changing relationships between individuals and teams. Formal evidence of culture change and a corresponding improvement in outcomes is limited, although (in line with integration) this does not mean that 'culture' is not a vital factor. Leadership is thought to make an important contribution to the creation and sustainability of a desired (or not so welcome) culture.

Culture, and in particular, cultural differences and clashes between professional groups and their organisational ways of doing business, has been raised within numerous studies of integration. Two helpful models to understand the types of issues that are connected with culture are those by Schein (2010) and Johnson and Scholes (2001). Schein proposes that culture can be seen as operating on three levels – values (ideologies or charters), artefacts (physical manifestations such as dress code, company reports and environment) and assumptions (thought processes, feelings and behaviour). These levels can be further differentiated into three domains in which organisational culture is enacted – *patients* (or service users, in our terms), *people* and *place* (Gale *et al.* 2014). Table 8.2 provides an interpretation of this framework in relation to an integrated care initiative. The artefacts listed can by themselves provide practical challenges to the running of an integrated care initiative. As importantly, though, they can signify (or be interpreted as signifying) a deeper assumption about the services and professional groups that contribute to an integrated care initiative. For example, if one professional has greater access to funding and time to undertake development, this can be seen as a symbol of how this profession is seen as more important.

Johnson and Scholes developed the 'cultural web' as an accessible framework to present the symbolic, political and structural aspects that influence the overall 'paradigm' or ways of thinking within an organisation. Such 'deep thinking' is key to how organisations will interpret and therefore respond to opportunities and circumstances that they encounter, and understanding the paradigm can help to explain why stakeholders can see a similar problem or solution so differently. Figure 8.1 provides an overview of key questions that can be deployed in order to explore the paradigms within an integrated care initiative.

Table 8.2: Observable artefacts commonly encountered in an integrated care initiative

Domain	Example of common artefacts within an integrated care initiative
Service users	Terminology: tenants, patients, service users or clients are but a few of the terms that are used within these sectors
	Relationship: service users in housing have to sign a legal tenancy agreement, whereas in health there may be no signed care plan
	Charging: healthcare is largely free, whereas charging applies in social care and housing
People engaged in delivering a service	Staff dress: uniform commonly worn by health staff that differentiates between them and non-health staff, and between different health disciplines
	Terms & Conditions: staff may be entitled to different holidays or opportunities for learning and development
	Payment: salary differentials lead to distinct variations in holidays, cars and housing
Place in which services are delivered	Location: are service users required to come to a discrete building or are they supported in their own home?
	Use of building: if a discrete building, is this shared with other services and organisations?
	Standard of building: is the building in a good state of repair and designed for the service in question?
	Facilities for staff: are there different expectations on office and desk arrangements, and facilities for refreshments?

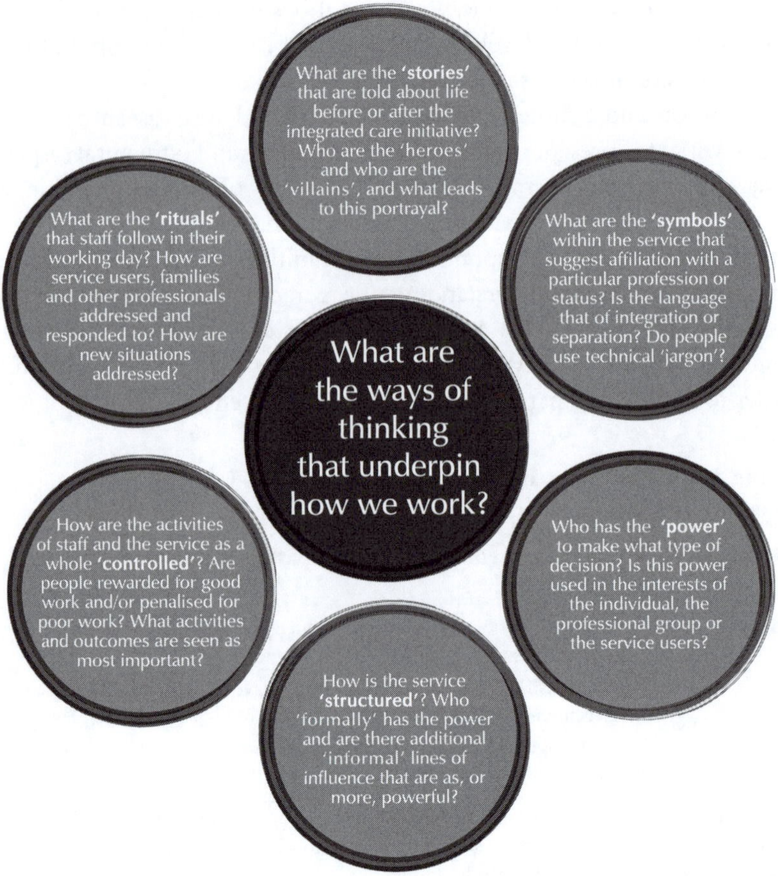

What are the **'stories'** that are told about life before or after the integrated care initiative? Who are the 'heroes' and who are the 'villains', and what leads to this portrayal?

What are the **'rituals'** that staff follow in their working day? How are service users, families and other professionals addressed and responded to? How are new situations addressed?

What are the **'symbols'** within the service that suggest affiliation with a particular profession or status? Is the language that of integration or separation? Do people use technical 'jargon'?

What are the ways of thinking that underpin how we work?

How are the activities of staff and the service as a whole **'controlled'**? Are people rewarded for good work and/or penalised for poor work? What activities and outcomes are seen as most important?

Who has the **'power'** to make what type of decision? Is this power used in the interests of the individual, the professional group or the service users?

How is the service **'structured'**? Who 'formally' has the power and are there additional 'informal' lines of influence that are as, or more, powerful?

Figure 8.1: Key aspects of a cultural web within an integrated care initiative

What interventions can positively respond to these aspects?

We have presented *professions, skills and knowledge* and *culture* separately to provide clarity about what the terms refer to, and the particular issues that they have been shown to lead to within integrated care initiatives. It will be clear, though, that there is a strong connection between these aspects. For example, the extent to which professional training has incorporated working with other disciplines will partly determine skills in communicating effectively, and professional cultures influencing people's willingness to participate in joint development sessions. The interventions that can be taken therefore need to be sensitive to the three aspects, and can seek to respond to one or more of them simultaneously.

Furthermore, the interventions themselves can interact, and should be deployed on the basis of the issues identified when initially planning the integrated care initiative (see Chapter 2) and emerging evaluation findings (see Chapter 9). The four staff-based interventions we will be focusing on in the sections that follow are supervision, inter-professional learning, team working, and communities of practice (CoPs).

How can we use supervision within an integrated care initiative?

Supervision of practice is a core requirement for all health and care professions to retain their professional status. Employers should also provide it for non-professional practitioners as a means to promote good practice and to ensure good quality of care.

Supervision has been shown to provide a number of important supports to staff members (Carpenter *et al.* 2012):

- providing an opportunity to reflect on aspects of practice about which the individual feels less confident

- considering options for intervention including the opportunities presented by new treatment and support

- receiving professional advice and having informed discussions about unfamiliar and high-risk situations

- offering a forum in which they can express the emotional impact of their jobs and the impacts that their decisions may have on the lives of others

- making staff feel valued and nurtured as individual professionals and practitioners.

It has also been shown to have benefits for the service through improving job satisfaction, encouraging engagement and commitment, and helping reduce staff turnover. These benefits for individual staff and for the service are also then likely to have benefits for service users through improving the consistency and quality of the service offered.

The importance of supervision is in many ways heightened within an integrated setting as staff will be based with professionals and practitioners from different disciplines and may not have a more senior or indeed other colleague from the same background. This can reduce the opportunity for peer support (which can also help with the aspects listed above), and contribute to the feelings of isolation and professional dilution mentioned above (see also Table 8.3).

Table 8.3: Types of supervision

Type of supervision	Usually completed by...	Purpose
Managerial	Supervisor with accountability and authority	Review their performance Set priorities/objectives in line with the organisation's objectives and service needs Identify training and continuing development needs
Clinical	Experienced clinician/ practitioner of same background	Reflect on and review their practice Discuss individual cases in depth Change or modify their practice and identify training and continuing development needs
Professional	Experienced clinician/ practitioner of same professional background	Review professional standards Keep up to date with developments in their profession Identify professional training and continuing development needs Ensure that they are working within professional codes of conduct and boundaries
Inter-professional	No common arrangement	Reflect on the individual's experience of working within an integrated care initiative Identify training and development needs relating to inter-professional practice Discuss opportunities to improve integrated care received by service users and their families

The terms 'clinical' and 'professional supervision' are often used interchangeably (see Table 8.3), and in many (but not all) cases will be provided through the same process. 'Managerial supervision' is again linked, but through its focus on organisational objectives and performance of the staff member in relation to these, it has a more distinct focus. Within an integrated care initiative there is also another aspect of practice that needs to be considered and incorporated within a supervision structure – that of inter-professional working. The key stakeholders, functions and elements of supervision have been brought together in a 4×4×4 model of supervision (SCIE 2013) that incorporates:

- four *stakeholders* – service user, professional/practitioner, organisation and partnership
- four *functions* – management, support, mediation and development
- four *elements* – experience, reflection, analysis and action planning.

There is no single way to provide supervision within an integrated care initiative, and the key issue is that all the elements outlined in Table 8.3 are available to all professionals and practitioners. For example, if the person's line manager is of a different profession, there can be a separation between managerial and clinical/professional, with the latter being provided by an individual within the same service, from a different part of the same organisation or, indeed, from another organisation (see Case example 8.1). Group supervision is another option, and whilst developed in uni-professional settings, there is increasing evidence of the benefits of restorative supervision for both the supervisee and supervisor (see Chapter 4).

Case example 8.1: Occupational therapy supervision

Understanding the difference between professional accountability and operational line management was a breakthrough moment in Aneurin Bevan's Health Board, freeing occupational therapists (OTs) to work wherever they needed to work under the day-to-day direction of a team manager who could be from any agency or profession. The focus from within the Health Board's occupational therapy service shifted away from the protection of the existing organisational structure to the creation of a professional structure to support OTs, regardless of where they worked, to access professional supervision, annual appraisal, and training and development. Within new models of integrated service delivery, OTs remain professionally accountable to the most senior OT in their organisation, but are increasingly being deployed into teams to be managed on a day-to-day basis by an operational team manager. The creation of a very strong professional identity, which upholds a focus on occupation, is at the core of what makes OTs different from other professional groups. This was critical in enabling OTs to grow in skill and knowledge, with the confidence that they can perform their roles independently whilst completely supported by a robust governance framework.

What does this case example tell us?

» It is possible to separate out line management and professional supervision and development so that they are delivered through different processes and people.

» Moving away from the traditional structure led to a renewal of professional identity and purpose.

Source: Kelly (2015)

What contribution can training and development make?

Providing training and development opportunities are an obvious way to support staff members who will be working within an integrated care initiative to develop the skills, knowledge and values that have been identified through their supervision and appraisals. Within the field of integration there has been particular interest in the potential of inter-professional approaches to such training and development. Inter-professional education (or IPE as it is often shortened to) is differentiated by the expectation that participants will not only learn alongside those from other professions and functions, but also that they will actively learn through interactions with each other (see Table 8.4). Much interest and research in inter-professional learning to date has related to undergraduate training, but there is also a growing body of evidence regarding its deployment within continuing professional development. Case example 8.2 demonstrates how theories of education can be practically applied:

- Locality teams were expected to produce a real business case to respond to a local priority for integration (*experiential learning*).

- Flexibility was built within the programme to enable participants to identify additional/alternative areas of learning (*adult learning*).

- There were multiple opportunities for reflection through action learning sets, personal diaries, team reviews and individual development sessions (*reflective practice*).

- Participants were expected to work in their teams to undertake work-based tasks in between block teaching days at the university (*collaborative learning*).

- There was an emphasis on professionals within teams sharing knowledge and skills and encouragement to explore differences as well as areas of overlap (*social learning*).

Table 8.4: Different types of learning

Type of learning	Description	Scenario example
Uni-professional	Professionals learn in isolation from other professional groups	Updates for physiotherapists on the latest developments in physical therapy Attendance of an OT at a national occupational therapy conference Training for home carers on manual handling
Multi-professional	Professionals learn alongside other professional groups	Presentation on new areas of policy and legislation that could affect many professionals and practitioners in the service Briefing on new information-sharing protocols within the organisation
Inter-professional	Professionals learn with, from and about each other	Adult safeguarding training in which different professions participate in interactive sessions based around case studies People-centred care planning in which service users talk to groups about their experiences, and there is group reflection on their insights

In designing an inter-professional learning opportunity it is important to follow a mapping process similar to the one followed in Chapter 2 for the integrated care initiative as a whole, with expected outcomes clearly identified along with the learning opportunities that would enable these to be achieved. The framework outlined earlier can be a helpful structure to think through and set expected outcomes in relation to the competences of staff members. A helpful means to frame the learning objectives is that provided by Kirkpatrick and Kirkpatrick (2007), which is adapted below, in a series of related questions:

- *Experience:* Do participants report having found the learning opportunity interesting, relevant and enjoyable?

- *Learning:* Did participants gain the expected knowledge and skills, and were these retained after the development opportunity?

- *Behaviour:* Did this additional knowledge and skills lead to a change in their professional and inter-professional practice?

- *Impact:* Has any change in behaviour contributed to the achievement of the expected benefits for service users and carers, financial efficiency and improving population health?

Inter-professional learning can be provided through more formal and discrete sessions (see Case examples 8.2 and 8.3). However, there are numerous other means to provide development opportunities that can positively engage professionals and practitioners, which may not require additional resources and external facilitators. For example, opportunities for different team members to present a case study of a service user they are supporting can be an excellent structure to demonstrate the work of the different professions. If this includes time for others to contribute their thoughts regarding existing challenges faced by the service user, this can improve the integrated care that they receive. Service users may also find such sessions illuminating and constructive, and can participate directly in such reflective learning. This does, of course, need to be well structured to avoid being tokenistic or, worse, distressing for the service user. Shadowing other professionals and practitioners is another inexpensive but informative opportunity for understanding more about the work of others. Debriefing from complaint investigations and sharing compliments provides insights regarding how service users and carers are experiencing the care provided, and the potential for collaborative action planning to respond to weaknesses and to build on strengths.

Although outwith the focus of this book, it is worth noting the rich learning opportunity that an integrated care initiative can provide for undergraduates and other trainees. Providing such opportunities is vital if we are to enable the professionals of the future to be able to work together successfully, and there is evidence that students can take on negative stereotypes of other professions during their training that inhibits their willingness to then work with other disciplines. Students are also often good at challenging our ways of thinking through bringing a fresh pair of eyes and the latest thinking in practice!

Case example 8.2: The Integrated Care Development Programme (ICDP)

The ICDP was a continuing inter-professional educational programme for health and social care managers and commissioners. Multi-professional strategic teams from a single locality participated in university and workplace-based learning activities centred on the development of an integrated business plan to address a local priority for improvement. These learning activities included taught sessions exploring research and theory, group discussions and presentations, challenge events in which external stakeholders critiqued draft plans, and reflective exercises.

The evaluation used participant self-assessment, semi-structured interviews and group discussions to assess the achievement of expected impacts on the participants, their organisations and partnerships, and patient/service user outcomes. The findings indicate that whilst those employed in management and commissioning roles had considerable experience of working across professional and agency boundaries, they derived individual benefits from a workplace IPE programme. The principles of design and delivery developed in pre-registration and clinician/practitioner IPE courses also applied to those working at a more strategic level. Organisational impacts were reported, but six months post-programme, evidence was not yet available of significant improvements in patient outcomes and/or financial efficiencies. Individual motivation, team dynamics and support from line managers all affected the extent to which individual and organisational impacts were achieved.

What does this case example tell us?

» Adult learners respond to education that is based around the real tasks and pressures that they encounter, and to flexibility in the activities provided.

» Inter-professional issues are also present at more senior management levels, and can be positively addressed through shared learning opportunities.

» Alongside individual commitment and ability, more contextual factors such as support from organisations influence engagement and learning.

Source: Miller et al. (2014)

Case example 8.3: 'Sliding Doors'

NHS Education for Scotland, the Scottish Social Services Council and a learning and development consultancy developed the Sliding Doors resources. These aimed to support health and social care staff in understanding a new model of care that valued older people as community assets, ensured their voices were heard, and supported them to enjoy full and positive lives in their own home or a community setting. The workshop commenced with participants considering what a 'good life' meant to them. Identifying their personal outcomes early in the session encouraged participants to have a personal connection with what followed. An actor portraying 'Maggie', an older woman with dementia, diabetes and depression, and 'Iain', her husband, interrupted the discussion. Participants gained an insight through the unfolding drama into what was important to Iain and Maggie – what made a 'good life' for them. This made a connection between the participants and the actors. The participants then worked in groups to discuss what they had learned about Iain and Maggie, and what they needed to know and do as professionals to support Iain and Maggie's expressed 'good life'. The drama then continued. Two years passed – Maggie was less able, and Iain had to go into hospital for a minor operation. This change represented a turning point: how Iain and Maggie's lives moved forward from here would depend on the responses and actions of everyone around them.

The film 'Sliding Doors' (directed by Peter Howitt in 1998) shows two possible futures for a young woman. In one, she catches a tube train, meets a man, and finds love and fulfilment. In the other, she misses the train and her life continues as a struggle. The chance event of catching the train or not – determined by the 'sliding doors' of the tube train closing – is a turning point for the possible future she will follow. In the workshop, 'sliding doors' acts as a metaphor to describe participants' potential to positively influence people's lives. It promotes awareness of how their decisions and actions as professionals affect other people going forward, and causes them to reflect on whether they support them to 'live the life they want to live' or not. This requires understanding of what is important to individual people at specific times in their lives. The aim of this exploration of the turning points in Iain and Maggie's lives is to help participants to understand the cultural and practice shifts they need to make as professionals. Iain and Maggie directly challenge them towards the end of the workshop to make two or three key commitments as people with sufficient influence to help ensure their future stays close to what is important to them in their 'good life'.

What does this case example tell us?

» Putting the lives of service users and carers at the heart of IPE makes the learning relevant and engaging to professionals and practitioners.

» More creative methods such as drama can be used to illustrate alternative ways of thinking and practising.

Source: Walker and Gillies (2014)

How can we develop good team working?

Most professionals and practitioners operate as a team, and indeed, many are part of several teams at the same time. The centrality of teams to our work, and the contribution that good team working can make to achieving integrated care, has become increasingly recognised. This is also true for 'non'-integrated teams, although in reality, most teams within the health, social care and housing sectors will contain more than one profession and/or practitioner discipline. This includes senior management teams that will often have members from a financial and human resources (HR) background as well as a management and/or clinical or other professional background. When teams work well they are thought to lead to greater efficiency and effectiveness, and to be key facilitators of 'safe' services through open communication and shared problem-solving. Teams are also promoted on the basis that they will provide a more enjoyable and enriching work environment for the staff concerned, and so improve motivation and retention. There is some evidence to support these positive views (see Table 8.5), and also the contrary perspective, that dysfunctional teams are often highlighted as contributing to examples of poor, or indeed abusive, care.

Table 8.5: Summary of evidence of integrated teams

Beneficiaries	Summary of evidence
Service users and families	There is evidence that multi-disciplinary teams have positive impacts for cancer patients (including better care planning, improved satisfaction and longer survival times) and within mental health services (including reductions in severity of symptoms, fewer compulsory admissions and a better social situation). There are not always positive impacts reported, though, with examples of service users reporting that integrated teams were not easy to access or respectful in their approaches
Professionals and practitioners	Positive experiences of being part of a team can lead to improved job satisfaction, lower levels of stress and reduced injuries and sickness
Organisations	Teams can contribute to a reduction in errors and near-misses, and can support more enabling models of care that are based outside of institutional settings. Evidence regarding the cost-effectiveness of such teams is mixed, though, with examples of them being assessed as leading to better outcomes and lower costs, but also higher costs with no improvement in outcomes

Source: Jelphs, Dickinson and Miller (2016)

A key issue is that simply labelling a group of individuals a 'team' does not automatically enable them to work together successfully as one. This is often paraphrased as the divide between 'real' versus 'pseudo' teams, with real teams being described as 'comprised of [a] small, manageable number of members with an appropriate mix of skills and expertise, who are committed to a meaningful purpose and have collective responsibility to achieve performance objectives and outcomes' (Harris *et al.* 2013, p.22). Much of the work on teams in the UK has been based on the pioneering work of Michael West and colleagues at Aston University on the English NHS. Their work highlighted both the benefits of 'real' teams but also the damage caused by 'pseudo' teams. From their research and others exploring this field, it is possible to highlight a number of key issues that need to be considered when introducing or strengthening teams within an integrated care initiative. Interestingly, whilst the final arrangements and logistics may differ, the principles behind them apply to teams in any setting or service (see Figure 8.2 and Case example 8.4).

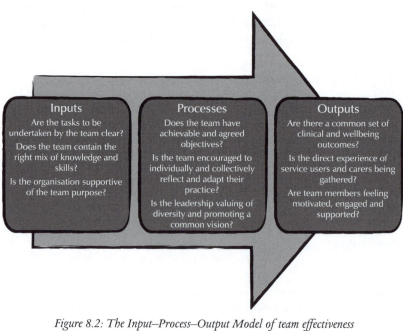

Figure 8.2: The Input–Process–Output Model of team effectiveness
Source: West and Lyubovnikova (2013)

Case example 8.4: Team working development in a fictional homeless scenario

The complex needs service undertook an evaluative review of its work that highlighted a number of key issues regarding team work in the service:

» Due to the 24-hour nature of the work and the shift patterns that were in operation, there were few opportunities for team members to meet as a whole.

» Whilst all staff members saw their overall purpose as being to support homeless people to improve their wellbeing and independence, there was a lack of agreement regarding the objectives that sat beneath these high-level aspirations, for example the point when the service user would be ready/ expected to leave the service.

» In addition to being part of the complex needs team, the practitioners were also members of inter-agency teams developed around individual service users. There was feedback from both staff and external stakeholders that these teams did not always function that well.

In view of the evidence regarding the importance of teams within integrated care initiatives, it was agreed to make developing their team work a key priority for the next 12 months. A simple electronic survey was developed mirroring the aspects of the Input–Process–Output Model (see earlier), and circulated to all the team members. A whole service event was arranged, with cover being provided to enable all staff members (including those who work at night) to attend. The results of the survey were shared, and a series of interactive group sessions used to jointly reflect and respond to the findings. Alongside this more internal focused activity, the service's steering committee was informed of the issues regarding the inter-agency teams. The committee contained representatives from these key agencies and decided to undertake joint work to strengthen collaboration within these temporary teams. This included bringing various professionals and practitioners together in development sessions to consider scenarios based on situations previously faced by service users.

Can communities of practice make a positive contribution?

Much of the current thinking and practice regarding communities of practice (CoPs) arises from the work of Wenger and colleagues. They originally proposed the term to describe the process through which 'novices' engaged in 'situated learning' to reflect that this involved much more than simply acquiring knowledge, but also socialisation and identity of development. They subsequently redefined it to reflect the engagement of groups of individuals in creating and sharing knowledge, and suggested that they could and should be actively developed by organisations to support improvement (see Wenger, McDermott and Snyder 2002). They suggest three key characteristics of CoPs – *mutual engagement* (interaction with each other, developing relationships and negotiating meaning), *joint enterprise* (undertaking similar tasks, common opportunities to influence and producing joint outputs) and *shared repertoire* (the stories, artefacts, words and rituals that are created). Reviews of their impacts on practice indicate that they can have positive benefits in relation to implementing new processes and technology, facilitating knowledge transfer, completing basic training, and reducing professional isolation.

There is not a recommended size or membership for CoPs to work effectively, and different methods of communication and engagement between members (e.g. workshops, seminars, social media groups) can be effective (or not) depending on the purpose and context of the CoP. It is clear, though, that simply calling a network of people a CoP will not lead to one being experienced in practice.

CoPs are often uni-professional or within a single organisation, and in such circumstances can be a barrier to inter-professional working due to the strong relationships and shared knowledge between members acting as a barrier to the inclusion of those outside of the CoP. This does not mean that they should be disbanded, or that members of an integrated care initiative should be prohibited from participating in such CoPs. Indeed, withdrawing from established CoPs could lead to members of the service losing vital updates and connections within their professions or areas of interest. It is important, though, to map out the existing CoPs, to consider the benefits of connecting their work and assessing the risks to inter-professional working of their inherent boundaries. Individuals who are members of different CoPs can act as key boundary spanners for this process (see Chapter 4). Multi-professional and multi-organisational

CoPs can also be developed (perhaps through expansion of existing ones with a narrower membership) as part of an integrated care initiative (see Case examples 8.5 and 8.6).

Case example 8.5: Communities of practice (CoPs) for those working with the multiply excluded

The Multiple Exclusion CoP programme was developed to explore if CoPs could overcome fragmentation in services and staff feeling out of their depth due to uni-professional training and experience. Five CoPs were established in different localities with a small budget for housekeeping and facilitation support. Each was expected to have between 6 and 12 members that represented the housing, criminal justice, social care and health professions working with this user group. They met monthly to discuss anonymised case studies presented by their members. There was also an online forum to share information between the CoPs, with further support from the research team to identify relevant evidence and policy documents.

The CoPs seemed effective in building collaborative networks. They provided an opportunity to discuss the challenges that they all individually faced without the pressure of having to represent, or indeed defend, the interests of their separate agencies. Key aspects to these positive impacts were the use of the case studies, the opportunity for 'face-to-face' contact, and the sharing of evidence through the researchers. They were not sure that this positive experience would lead to improved outcomes for service users in the short term due to the wider context in which the services were operating and their limited membership.

What does this case example tell us?

» CoPs can provide a forum in which professionals and practitioners from different agencies and backgrounds can share experiences and insights.

» The common motivation was to improve the lives of a marginalised group through better inter-professional and inter-agency working.

» Spending time together with structured activities helps remove barriers on a micro level, but these remain on a macro level.

Source: Cornes et al. (2014)

Case example 8.6: Communities of practice (CoPs) and primary care improvement

To support the identification, management and treatment of patients with chronic kidney disease (CKD) in primary care, this project involved 19 general practices creating improvement teams. Based on the CoP principles, these included a GP, a practice manager and a practice nurse who were supported by an external facilitator from the research team. The latter included nephrologists, management academics and analysts. Team members in the practices had different motivations for participating, including an overall passion for learning and improvement, an interest in CKD in particular, and the potential to gain more income through better achievement of quality standards. It was also hoped that the practises would form a wider CoP during the project.

The multi-professional nature of the teams was seen largely as positive, and their shared commitment to their practise and patients provided a common focus. In the smaller practices there was better engagement from other practice staff who also often attended the CoP meetings, whereas in the larger practices it seemed more difficult to get other practice members on board due to a lack of identification with the team's work and other demands on their time through other initiatives. The CoP between the practices was less successful, with limited participation in teleconferences and an online community. Key factors that contributed to this were thought to be competition between the practices to be 'the best' in their area, and a tradition of uni-professional networks as the vehicles for information sharing.

What does this case example tell us?

» CoPs worked well within smaller services as a means to bring together professionals and practitioners through face-to-face meetings around a shared interest.

» CoPs based on virtual meetings and online forums were less successful due to rivalries and a lack of shared connection with those from different professions and services.

Source: Kislov, Walshe and Harvey (2012)

Chapter 9

Working with Processes and Systems

Throughout the book so far we have emphasised the people element of integrated care, and the importance of engaging service users, family carers and professionals and practitioners in the development and delivery. There is also, though, a role for systems and processes to support integration to become 'real' and to hardwire it within the local context. Indeed, without integrated systems and processes, well-meaning attempts to integrate services are at risk of withering on the vine. This is particularly the case when the person or people who initially lead it leave for pastures new and the initial vision and inspiration is lost (see Chapter 10). Having integrated systems and processes can change the behaviour of professionals, makes integration the default position, makes people's lives easier, and reduces the risk of the initiative failing.

A wide range of systems and processes can be developed to support and drive integrated initiatives. No one approach will achieve integration, but we suggest that there are four key areas that you will want to consider:

- What systems and processes will support prioritisation of services across the population?

- What systems and processes will support coordination across organisations?

- What systems and processes will support sharing of data and information between professionals and between professionals and individuals?

- What systems and processes will support quality and probity?

A word about IT

We are all aware that a huge issue for people seeking to integrate across organisations are the multi and various IT systems in use in different parts of the system. These are often incompatible, which reduces opportunities for data sharing, and non-accessible, so integrated teams may not be able to access each other's data. In an ideal world there would be a single IT system for all agencies in an integrated initiative. Some people may have the opportunity to commission a new IT system for their integrated initiative, although this is unlikely to be the case for most. This chapter therefore focuses on those systems and processes that can be put in place without the luxury of an aligned IT system.

A useful lesson from Wales is set out in Case example 9.1: the Single Point of Access (SPA) pilots.

Case example 9.1: IT and practical solutions

On reflection, the SPA pilots would have benefited from following an integrated social services and health information system – in the words of one of our IT experts, 'the holy grail'. Our response has been to 'accept and adapt'; we do not sweat over those things which we have no control...

We have kept our focus on our vision for SPA, with each site finding the best interim solution, albeit much to the frustration of our IT leads, who would prefer one approach. The differences between systems is inevitably an impediment in the short term – therefore a local interim solution was needed, a solution that lends itself to an easy transition, when we have one integrated system.

Sadly, until that time, the true benefit of SPA to save duplication and hence realise efficiencies will not be realised. We are now well versed in the 'art of compromise', but without losing our principles and vision.

A word about joint finance

As with IT systems, in an ideal world we would have pooled budgets for any integrated initiative. Aligning or pooling budgets helps overcome the fragmentation issues inherent in the current systems, can achieve better value for money by reducing duplication, and arguably would ideally be the starting place for any integrated initiative. However, the current finance systems of organisations involved in health and care are not set up to support integrated working and in some cases, in fact, work against working in partnership.

Recent legislation has promoted pooling budgets at a strategic level. For example, in England, clinical commissioning groups (CCGs) and local authorities have been required to operate a pooled budget as part of the Better Care Fund, and in Scotland, legislation sets out what has to go into a pooled budget from the health board and local authority, what is excluded, and what may be included. An *aligned* budget involves two or more partners working together to jointly consider their budgets and to align their activities to deliver agreed aims and outcomes, whilst retaining complete accountability and responsibility for their own resources. A *pooled* budget is an arrangement where two or more partners make financial contributions to a single fund to achieve specified and mutually agreed aims. It is a single budget, managed by a single host, with a formal partnership or joint funding agreement that sets out aims, accountabilities and responsibilities (see Case Study 9.2).

When considering your integrated initiative, you may not be in a position to enter into pooled budget arrangements. You should therefore consider whether an aligned budget approach is possible. Creating this arrangement is often initially much simpler and may be more appropriate where partnership working is at an early stage.

Case example 9.2: Pooled budget for equipment

In Herefordshire they have pooled budgets for managing adaptations and equipment to help people to live independently at home after they have come out of hospital, or to support disabled children at school. Accessed by district nurses, occupational therapists and social workers, the service enables faster and efficient use of equipment across the county, providing improved health and social care. Most equipment is now delivered and fitted within two days of the original request. And there are significant savings on management costs, and from joint purchasing of equipment.

What does this case example tell us?

» Pooled budgets used appropriately can be an enabler of more responsive services and improved outcomes for service users.

What systems and processes will support prioritisation of services across the population?

The accurate identification of individuals appropriate for an integrated care intervention is crucial to the success of the approach. Without a reliable method of stratifying people into risk groups, services may be targeted at those who do not need it, and potentially miss those who do. Predictive risk tools are increasingly being employed in the NHS and more recently within social care. Risk stratification can be used to identify people who would benefit most from targeted interventions (known as case finding), and can be used to allocate resources across a population, and for performance management and evaluation purposes. For example, it could divide a population, such as a general practice patient list, into different levels of risk for a specified outcome, such as unscheduled admissions to hospital.

NHS England (2015) defines case finding as 'a systematic or opportunistic process that identifies individuals' (e.g. people with chronic obstructive pulmonary disease from a general practice list to identify them for a flu vaccination).

Much of the risk stratification approach is currently focused on health data. However, if it is possible to add certain social care data into a 'risk engine', then case finding and risk stratification can support an approach that aims to identify the health and social care determinants of risk of admission to hospital, or other adverse social care outcomes, for example permanent admission to a care home or those at risk of social isolation.

Case example 9.3: Risk stratification in Enfield

The London Borough of Enfield wanted to identify those at risk of needing intensive social care and those at risk of social isolation so they could put them in touch with voluntary sector organisations as part of their integrated offer. They used the Nuffield PARR-30 (people at risk of readmission) algorithm, and populated it with primary care data from GPs and secondary care data from acute trusts on a monthly basis, as well as adding in adult social care data. The GPs receive a list of their own patients categorised into very high, high, moderate and low risk. Only they can identify people and only their own patients; everyone else can only see aggregate reports. Data-sharing issues were addressed by asking patients for informed consent.

What does this case example tell us?

>> Risk stratification is an approach that can utilise data from across the system to identify individuals who could benefit from preventative services and approaches.

Risk stratification can be a complex, sophisticated approach using an online 'risk engine'. There are many risk stratification tools available, most of which focus on health risk stratification. Nuffield has produced a guide for people seeking to procure a risk stratification too (see the Resources section at the end of this book). However, risk stratification can also be used more informally within a multi-disciplinary team to identify the issues that might put individuals at risk and to discuss how they could be supported.

What systems and processes will support coordination across organisations?

The systems that enable coordination across organisations are central to an effective integrated initiative. They are the systems that ensure that the user is at the centre of the system, and that their outcomes are the ones on which professionals focus.

Case management is the generic term for a range of processes that involve a targeted, community-based and proactive approach to care. It involves assessment and care planning, care coordination and accurate case finding to ensure patients with highly complex and multiple conditions receive effective support. The processes involved are explored in more detail below.

Assessment and care planning

Developing a joint assessment and care planning approach is key when working in an integrated initiative. An approach must be designed that meets the statutory needs of each agency, but more fundamentally ensures that the service user is placed at the centre of the process, and only has to provide their information once. This is an area where technology can really help so that assessments and care plans can be completed with users and then be shared with relevant colleagues quickly and easily. Single/joint, holistic or community-based assessment processes have been developed in a range of areas. The challenge is to ensure that these are used, and that professionals trust the assessments made by their colleagues.

Single point of referral or access

Providing one point of entry into the service, irrespective of where someone might 'present' themselves, is fundamental to ensuring a focus on individuals. Many integration initiatives have developed this approach, and have maximised the use of available technology (see Case example 9.4). In Cornwall, for example, they developed a 'community line' that is manned by volunteers and provides a trusted link between local multi-disciplinary teams, key workers and local resources. In South Devon and Torbay they are developing a unified call centre, services directory, e-hub and website.

Case example 9.4: Single Point of Access (SPA) for mental health in Shropshire

Bromford is a social business operating across Central England that provides homes and support services to over 60,000 people. In 2007 the organisation worked with the primary care trust and Shropshire Council to develop an accommodation-based recovery project that would enable the step-down of acute patients discharged from hospital and residential care homes, and those returning from out-of-area placements. The scheme generated £1.7 million in savings in the first five years.

The accommodation offered contains seven individual flats and includes a community hub where tenants can access information and support to aid them in their recovery. Housing and support allocations are made through an SPA for mental health scheme operated across Shropshire. This means that all providers and practitioners work through one process that includes multi-agency joint assessments. Central to the success of the scheme has been the adoption of a 'one team' approach, working closely with the local foundation trust recovery team. It is based on strong multi-agency relationships, where everyone works as one team in the best interests of the service users, and liaises with a wide network of community agencies operating across the county. The partnership is strengthened through relationships that pay close attention to community and clinical risk, joining up assessments to create a more comprehensive understanding of the patient journey. The relationship plays to each other's strengths, enabling people to integrate into the community whilst their clinical needs are met.

What does this case example tell us?

» Developing an SPA underpinned by a multi-agency team approach around the needs of service users can enable people to integrate into the community as well as meet their health needs.

Care coordination

There is no single definition of care coordination, and it can mean different things in different places. The typical approach involves the role of a care coordinator, navigator or broker, whose job it is to help service users and carers navigate an often complex and overwhelming set of services and different providers. The concept of a care coordinator is different from other roles such as case managers and advocates because their focus is on *reducing* barriers to care.

Care coordinators can play a variety of roles depending on the context in which they are working. There are a wide range of models of care coordinator roles that offer a variety of services including assessment and care planning, coordination of care, phone support, home visits, liaison with medical and community services, and patient and care-giver education. They support people to use their personal budget, and provide information and advice if they are not eligible for support. Accountability for achieving outcomes with the user then lies with the care coordinator. The key aspect of the role is that it requires coordinators to advocate for the patient and to broker access to appropriate care as they transition across settings or providers.

Care coordination is often developed alongside a multi-disciplinary team approach, so that the care coordinator acts as the single point of contact, both for the individual and also for the providers and professionals on the team. Different levels of care coordination will be appropriate for different individuals, and support can range from a simple directory of services, a person having a named professional as a first point of contact with the health system, or a navigator responsible for coordinating health and social care for people with multiple, complex long-term conditions.

There are numerous potential benefits (see Case example 9.5) of having a single point of contact for coordinating care across providers, including the following:

• The individuals and their carers understand who to call in a crisis, and have a single, simple point of contact. Knowing there is someone to contact can significantly improve levels of confidence and emotional wellbeing.

- The service user is clear about who is ultimately responsible for coordinating their care.

- There is continuity in the provision of care services, so that individuals can build relationships with their care coordinators.

- Successful coordination can help avoid duplication in care, as care is managed by a single person rather than a system.

The type of person who acts as the care coordinator depends on the role they are expected to play. For example, individuals with less complex cases may have a care coordinator who is a volunteer, and who they only see once a month, whilst those who have very complex needs may have a coordinator who is a nurse or nurse practitioner, who they see once a week or once every two weeks. People who could act as care coordinators include volunteers, nurse practitioners, GPs, administrative staff and specially employed care coordinators who have a mix of clinical and administrative training.

Case example 9.5: Examples of care coordination approaches

Clinical navigators in Hertfordshire

Clinical navigators are based in the A&E department and assess people before admission. When hospital admission is not considered the best course of action, the clinical navigators offer guidance and advice about care in the community. When necessary, they also liaise with health, social care and voluntary services to arrange ongoing support for the person. Recent evaluation of the service shows that 81 per cent of people seen by a clinical navigator were not admitted to hospital, and were signposted to more appropriate services.

Care navigators in the London Borough of Greenwich

Care navigators (non-clinical) act as the central contact point for each service user, guide them through the various services, and ensure their personal plan is being followed. Once people have been identified as needing the service, the care navigator will listen to the patient or their carer to understand their individual needs. The team that the individual needs to help them then meets to solve as many of these complex problems as possible, and will often find innovative solutions. Each individual has a named professional who coordinates their integrated care plans, so that patients don't have to repeat their story to numerous professionals. As well as working directly with a number of high-risk individuals, the role of care navigators is also to raise awareness amongst GPs and other community and social care staff of the array of voluntary and community services in the borough that can contribute to the health and wellbeing needs of their patients and clients.

The care navigator service has access to a combined community/mental health record. It is located in the community and includes social workers as well as a health professional as the lead. A GP involved in the pilot said, 'The approach has really improved the experience of my patients. In one particular case, a patient who was attending A&E several times a week by ambulance has now only attended three times over the past three months when calling 111. Their housing issues have been sorted, they have received appropriate financial advice and support, their diabetes is much more controlled and their overall health has improved.'

In addition to care navigators, the role of *community navigators* is also emerging. These tend to be voluntary roles, which are focused on undertaking holistic assessments and signposting people to community support.

Voluntary care navigators in Kent

Voluntary Action within Kent manages the Care Navigation project, in partnership with Carers First. The care navigators will usually visit people in their homes and provide advice around a number of issues, including managing money and benefits, finding the right sort of home, maintaining and adapting homes to needs, planning the support needed, filling in forms, and going through an assessment process. The care navigators will also support people to make contact with other professional organisations and agencies.

What do these examples tell us?

» Navigator roles can be effective in guiding service users to more appropriate services.

Managed care networks (MCNs)

MCNs are integrated care networks that bring professionals together through a network approach. Operating on a local, regional or national basis, MCNs link practitioners across organisational boundaries to deliver care for a specific condition, care group or service. They promote virtual integration through collaborative working across care sectors within an agreed governance framework. MCNs are loose integration models that may have some form of governance (a manager or coordinator of the network), but the focus is on integrating service delivery. MCNs have been developing in Scotland, and extend the principles of clinical networks to health and social care, focusing on the equitable provision of high-quality services, by linked groups of professionals.

The success of the networks depends on building up trust between the partners and individual professionals working together (see Case example 9.6). At the operational level, trust develops as professionals and practitioners become accustomed to working together. To be successful, the partners in the network must share the same understanding of the network's goals.

Case example 9.6: Lincolnshire's MCN for mental health

The network comprises 44 full member organisations, including housing and social care representatives providing projects across Lincolnshire. In addition, it also comprises associate members – those groups and organisations that do not currently receive investment from the Mental Health Promotion Fund, but that remain as members to retain their links to the network. Lincolnshire's MCN for mental health aims to help people who have already experienced mental health problems, or who are having their first experience of mental illness. Members of the network have close links with each other to help people prevent, manage and recover from mental illness, so that people can enjoy the best possible quality of life.

What does this case example tell us?

> » MCNs can be a useful way for professionals to develop relationships and to continually improve services and outcomes for service users.

What systems and processes will support sharing of data and information between professionals and between professionals and individuals?

Being able to share data has many benefits. It supports integrated care records, caseload matching and risk stratification approaches. For users it can offer seamless pathways across services, only having to provide information once, improving planning and coordination of care, and ensuring that, in an emergency, the maximum amount of data about the individual is able to be shared.

However, data sharing is an area where many integrated initiatives fail, because there are so many perceived and real barriers to sharing data across (and sometimes within) organisations. The thing to remember is to focus on what you are trying to achieve – better outcomes for patients and users. In many cases, this relies on sharing information across internal boundaries and across organisations. However, it needs to be done with the knowledge and permission of individuals, as well as securely. The key issue is to balance the need to protect data with the need to share it, to achieve the best outcomes.

This section does not attempt to explore all the different challenges and potential solutions to share data across organisations as this is a huge area and many other sources are available to support data-sharing approaches. Instead, we suggest some questions that you and your colleagues from partner organisations could ask that will help shape your approach to developing a local set of shared data:

- What do you want to know? (Start with this, rather than starting with what you already collect.)

- What anecdotal data do you have? (For example, informal, emergent data.)

- What proxy indicators are available? Do you have any benchmark data, or data from providers?

- Do you understand who owns the data and how you might be able to share it?

- If data-sharing issues present a barrier, what is the minimum you can share?

- Do you understand the information governance rules?

- Can you work with providers to develop local datasets?

- How important is data collection and generation as part of the integrated initiative?

- Do you have the senior leadership and buy-in you need to make it happen?

- What local-level datasets are available already?

A fundamental underpinning of integrated initiatives is to develop multi-disciplinary working, whether that is by bringing different professionals together to contribute to a new approach, creating a formal team structure, or informally through multi-disciplinary team meetings or inter-professional networks (see Chapter 8). The suggestions below about the systems to enable data and information sharing are based on an assumption that multi-disciplinary team working in some form is, or will be, part of your integrated approach.

Record keeping

Developing integrated care records that can also be shared with users can enable much quicker support to be offered, with users not having to tell their story, and all members of a team having access to the same up-to-date information and data. Integrated record keeping enables care professionals to access the same quality, comprehensive and up-to-date information about an individual, and supports care coordination (see Case example 9.7).

Case example 9.7: Cheshire shared digital care record

Shared digital care records should allow care professionals to access the same quality, comprehensive and up-to-date information about an individual so they have a clear picture of their needs and can act quickly to support them – for instance, sharing information across a multi-disciplinary team to plan for hospital discharge. When fully developed, the shared digital record in Cheshire should include: primary care summary record, medication, diagnostic results and reports, clinical correspondence, summaries and assessments, key contacts, summary social care records and details of care plans and service providers, and details of community appointments and of care plans and services provided.

The information governance issues around such integrated records are currently unclear, but implied consent may be used as the most straightforward means of sharing data. Some methodologies do not need the data to be stored but bring the records together at the point they are required, and then remove the link immediately after. If you are considering developing an integrated record, you may want to seek advice on the information governance rules.

Patient held records (PHRs)

Some areas have developed PHRs, where the service user is given a copy of the record to keep, and to take to health appointments, to help manage healthcare tasks and communication. PHRs are formal and structured records that are given to patients to enable the continuity and quality of care. They include structured sections of patient and healthcare information and blank sections to enable patient note-taking and healthcare staff notes. This approach could usefully be shared within a multi-disciplinary team (see Case example 9.8).

Case example 9.8: Isle of Wight patient passport

On the Isle of Wight they have developed a system through which all parts of the health and care system can share information about patients and service users, through a 'patient passport' shared record system. This was developed using Eclipse, a web-based tool. It allows access to essential aspects of a person's medical records including clinical conditions, medications and allergies, blood results and investigations undertaken, as well as care plans. The patient passport puts the patient in control, allowing their healthcare plans to be implemented, and empowering them to decide which information is passed on to healthcare professionals. Appropriate professionals can securely access, within seconds, vital information from a person's medical records, enhancing the quality and safety of patient care.

What does this case example tell us?

» Giving service users control over their records is a powerful way of enabling them to have control over how their package of support is developed and what information is shared with services.

What systems and processes will support quality and probity?

Creating the governance system for an integrated care initiative can be complex and resource-intensive. It is important that the structures that you establish set the tone and act as a role model for the approach that you are establishing, but they need to be fit for purpose and not create a talking shop with a cast of thousands. Depending on the arrangements you are establishing, the governance structures might vary from a single integrated management team that meets weekly to a looser, multi-stakeholder steering group that might meet every couple of months.

The type of governance arrangements should reflect the depth of integration. If there is structural integration, for example where new teams are created from different organisations that will be managed within one organisation, or if there is a pooled budget, then you are likely to want robust structural governance arrangements such as a single management team. If you are overseeing a multi-disciplinary initiative where different organisations are contributing but are not being structurally integrated, then a steering group or board arrangement may be more appropriate. Some governance structures may already exist, such as a programme board, which your system will need to fit within.

Whatever arrangements you decide to put in place, you need to ensure that they move beyond acting as a discussion forum and coordination board, to become a forum where partners are held jointly accountable for delivery against the agreed performance metrics. It is vital to establish a sense of shared accountability; to do this, the governance structure should make it clear which organisations are accountable for each aspect of delivery, and the performance management metrics should be developed together and monitored regularly.

We suggest that there are three key elements to governance: structure, processes and actors (see Figure 9.1).

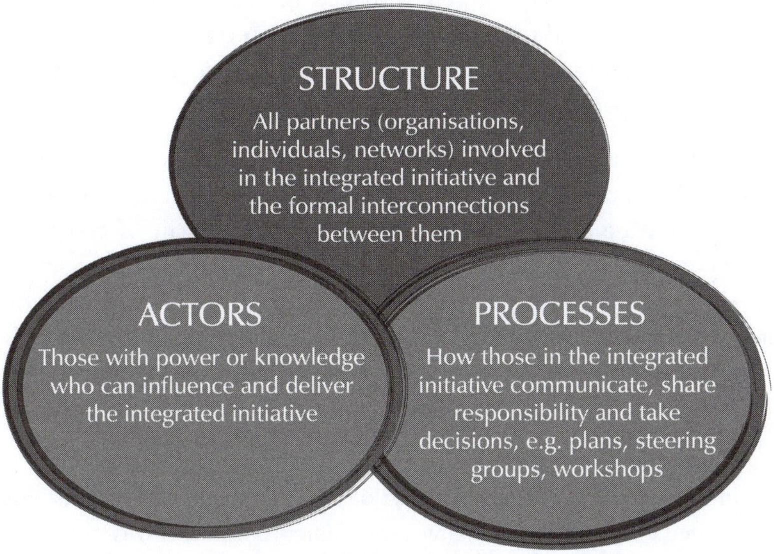

Figure 9.1: Governance of an integrated care initiative
Source: Vangen, Hayes and Cornforth (2015)

Structure: This determines who can influence the agenda and who can take important decisions and have the resources, power and legitimate authority to act and be accountable for its undertakings. In terms of structure it is important to decide whether you want a tight or loose structure – a tight structure of only a few people may exclude key stakeholders from influencing the collaboration's agenda but may be administratively more efficient. An open structure, where different organisations may attend, may make it harder to make decisions and to take things forward because it will be difficult to resolve differences between participants and to coordinate action. An open structure also means that it is difficult to establish clear lines of accountability. On the positive side, open structures encourage partners to contribute where there is a strong overlap between the goals of the collaboration and their own individual and organisational goals, so it is likely to create more commitment from organisations.

Processes: Governance processes include ways of communicating, sharing responsibility and taking decisions through actions such as developing plans, writing reports, monitoring progress, carrying out reviews, and holding workshops and seminars. The way in which the venue is chosen and the frequency by which partners meet and communicate can influence the way in which the integrated initiative works. For example, the meeting venue can have a big impact on governance. If meetings take place within the council chamber during the day, this sets expectations about how the integration is being managed, who is in the lead role, and what kind of people they expect to attend.

Actors: Within a governance system there are expectations that specific actors will direct, coordinate and allocate resources for the integration initiative, and be accountable for its activities. The chair of committees and steering groups can critically help or hinder others in their enactment of their leadership role, by the way in which the group is chaired, which may create an expectation that others look to them for leadership rather than creating a sense of shared accountability. The individuals with most influence are not always those in formal leadership roles (see the discussion in Chapter 4 on power bases.)

Within these parameters, there is a set of issues that you will need to think about when designing governance arrangements. Some of this may not be within your control, but it is worth asking the questions and challenging possible assumptions (e.g. about which organisation is the lead).

It will be up to you and your colleagues to decide which type of arrangements will work most effectively, and to keep the arrangements under review to ensure they are fit for purpose as the initiative develops.

To support your governance arrangements you will need to develop ways of understanding the performance of the initiative. In order to choose the right measures through which to manage quality, performance and progress in integrated care, there first needs to be a clear understanding of:

- the core aims of the integrated initiative
- the range of desired outcomes that should result from the initiative, focused on outcomes for the service users and their families
- the timeframe over which such outcomes can reasonably be expected to be achieved in order to understand which measurement categories actually have the potential to be improved
- how impact can be measured in a way that ensures attribution between the interventions developed and the outcomes observed
- the robustness of measures, so that they can imply actions to be undertaken for quality improvement purposes by managers and professionals, and to avoid perverse incentives

- simplicity and ease of measurement. Metrics would be usefully aligned to what people do anyway and the data they routinely collect, rather than asking them to collect new data

- a baseline measure collected so you can measure data over time, to enable you to understand trends and changes in performance.

Some of these issues may have been dealt with through your initial mapping work when developing the integrated initiative. If that work has not been done, agreeing what outcomes to measure will probably be a process of negotiation between the organisations and professions involved. Starting with what is already measured and collected is a pragmatic way to begin, but just measuring what is already collected may not reflect the outcomes that you are trying to achieve through integration. For example, you may not capture any data on how well you work together, but you may want to evaluate the impact of improved partnership working. A good starting point for a conversation is to agree on what you are trying to achieve and to then discuss how you might measure that. The concept of evidence often means different things to different professional groups, so this may be an ongoing, deliberative process rather than a one-off decision (see Case example 9.9).

Case example 9.9: Greenwich's approach to performance measurement

In Greenwich, we used an action learning approach that helped us to think creatively around what we wanted to measure and evaluate.

At the development stage, we really didn't know which features of the patient cohort would be the most useful to record in order to learn about, for example, unmet needs. On a number of occasions, we had to go back and refine what we were recording for the purposes of measuring outcomes.

To understand the engagement levels of the Greenwich Coordinated Care programme with the voluntary sector, we decided to capture which organisations were engaged, and tracked that as a percentage of the total number of relevant voluntary sector organisations. We were doing so well that we could start to apply more granularity and look at which services were commonly used from those organisations. More recently, the voluntary service director has even expressed her desire of wanting to understand which types of services (e.g. gardening clubs, advocacy and befriending) are most in demand under the big umbrella organisations such as Age UK and Mind.

We applied a qualitative as well as quantitative approach, as we felt that relying on quantitative data alone would not provide a complete picture. We have trialled some methods such as a staff questionnaire (via Survey Monkey) to assess engagement and learning from our Greenwich Coordinated Care meetings, although this did not provide us with any clear conclusions. We are therefore now developing the next questionnaire in partnership with a core group of staff as part of our action learning meetings, and hope that this will provide us with a useful insight.

What does this case example tell us?

» Recognise that this process will require a lot of refinement before you get it right.

» Once your measures become more refined, you will be able to gain further insight and act on it.

» Use qualitative information to support quantitative data. Don't get disheartened if an approach doesn't work, and keep trying.

Source: Better Care Fund (2015)

The checklist provided in Figure 9.2 is a quick outline of how you could approach the development of a performance measurement process.

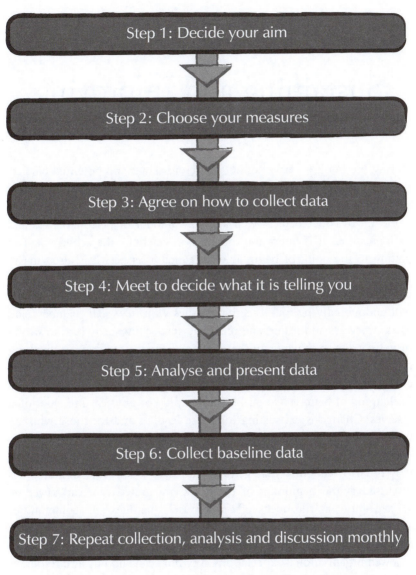

Figure 9.2: The seven steps – a quick approach to performance measurement

Chapter 10

Sustaining and Improving

During the book we have set out numerous issues and potential barriers that have to be overcome in order to successfully develop an integrated care initiative. Doing so will undoubtedly have involved considerable work for all concerned, as well as a fair amount of personal stress and time pressures. It is important therefore to celebrate the achievement of getting to the point of being able to launch a service. It is also vital to allow time for the new arrangements to settle in and provide a period of consolidation when the new ideas are tested out in practice. There will undoubtedly be initial teething issues with new staff members, job roles, processes and teams, and relatively small things may lead to strong responses due to the anxiety that we feel when we are doing something new. It is also a common experience for a major external crisis to come along just at the wrong time! And there will be a need for a collective 'recharging of batteries' to enable a rebuilding of physical and emotional reserves. Change is exhausting for those leading and for those who are participating.

Once the dust has settled and a degree of normality has been restored, it is time to recognise that getting launched is only the first step. As discussed at the beginning of the book, integrated care can never be a fixed entity as the needs of service users, families and communities are constantly changing. There will also be changes in context, with new opportunities and new demands from shifting national policies and renewed organisational expectations. Key financial and physical resources may be reduced or indeed added to, and the reliance of most integrated care initiatives on their professionals and practitioners brings in change due to personal lives and career opportunities. Furthermore, the harsh reality is that many integrated care initiatives are not sustained in the long term, and what can be seen as cutting-edge practice in one year may then be viewed as an unnecessary complication further down the line. The fault lines between health, social care and housing support run deep, and changes in financial environments and political priorities are inevitable.

In this chapter we consider what can be done to sustain and improve an integrated care initiative, and how we can positively respond to situations in which the initiative is no longer to continue. The following questions are explored:

- What are the common reasons that an integrated care initiative can lose its way?

- What can be done to ensure that an initiative continues to improve and be sustained?

- How is it best to ensure that the end of an initiative is not the end of integrated care?

What are the common reasons that an integrated care initiative can lose its way?

A decision to withdraw funding or to move to a new broader structure in which the integrated care initiative does not have a place is a common end point for integrated care initiatives. These can be due mainly to factors outwith the control or influence of the initiative, and may not be any reflection on the ability to achieve its aims and to deliver an excellent service. However, it is also possible for initiatives to lose the drive and purpose that they began with, and to become complacent about their ongoing need to improve. Overcoming the challenges to launch can seem like such an achievement that there is no further work to do when, in fact, they are best seen as a foundation on which further developments must then be crafted. If this happens, external stakeholders will be less likely to continue their support, particularly if previous senior champions have moved on. Furthermore, an integrated care initiative has no automatic right to survival, and failure to further adapt and develop should rightly question its future. Ensuring that there is a continued emphasis on improvement is therefore a key part of maintaining legitimacy and also ensuring that the initiative delivers value.

There are five common reasons that an integrated care initiative can start to lose its way:

Loss of focus: As set out earlier, there is often a key 'wicked issue' that leads to an integrated care initiative being considered. During the development phase there is the potential for stakeholders to add in other issues that may have some connections with the initial purpose, but which considerably broaden its reach and remit. This can be a good opportunity to increase impact, and may also be a necessity in terms of maintaining senior support. However, it can also dilute the overall aims, and lead to lack of clarity regarding the population to be served. Once initiatives are launched and being seen to make a difference, it is common for them to be asked to incorporate other services. These can be services that are seen as being in need of improvement and that would require considerable input to bring them up to speed with more dynamic and person-centred working. The initiatives may also be required to lead on new policy expectations regarding integrated care, even if these are with a different set of partners and populations.

Loss of relevance: Whilst wicked issues do, by their nature, last for a considerable length of time, this doesn't mean that they stand still. Indeed, it can be guaranteed that additional complexities will be added over time due to changes in demographics or local contexts. There may also be key changes in the organisations or services that the initiative works with, which means that previous arrangements are no longer fit for purpose. Or there may be new opportunities for integrated care that the initiative should respond to, or an innovation by another agency that addresses some of the needs. Failure to keep abreast with such changes in context, need and opportunity will decrease the relevance of the initiative to the problems that it wishes to sort out. These factors are not under the influence of the service, but a readiness to be aware of such fluctuations and willingness to respond to them is.

Loss of leadership: Integrated care initiatives are much more than their leaders, and (as set out in Chapter 4) leadership is much more than the person who takes on the role of senior manager or clinician. However, it is common that there will be one or several key individuals who are seen by both external stakeholders and staff members as being central to the running and development of an initiative. They are often instrumental to gathering support around a common vision, and act as boundary spanners, holding the different professional and practitioner groups and teams together. When these individuals move on, this can lead to a loss of confidence regarding the future of the initiative, and may result in past anxieties and even animosities returning to the surface.

Loss of engagement: Engagement of service users, carers and communities is a core part of establishing the purpose of a service. The promise of something new is a powerful motivator for people to become involved, as there is a tangible opportunity that things will change. The questions that can be asked are often quite exciting and far-reaching, as the final scope, and therefore its limitations, have not been established. It is also often easier to gather in additional funding or capacity to support engagement during the development phase, as its importance is generally recognised. Once an initiative is actually launched, the excitement and indeed engagement support may be lost, and this can lead to some fall-off in motivation and opportunity. The service may need to respond to concerns about its own practice and therefore lose some of its shine and start to be seen as part of the status quo. Similarly, staff engagement can be higher during the planning and transition stages as people are both inspired by the opportunity and also want to address any potentially negative impacts for their own work and career. Engagement of service users and staff remains, though, a key enabler of identifying and achieving future improvements.

Loss of resources: It is common for partnership agencies initially to be generous with resources in order to address the local wicked issue or to respond to the policy imperative. There may also be short-term funding available in order to set up these types of services. Over time, though, other priorities may emerge, or funding pressures become more difficult. The positive impact of the initiative may indeed contribute to this if it is possible to reduce concerns about the issue in question. Along with funding and the staffing and technological resources that it can enable is the issue of professionals and practitioners moving on to other jobs. This can be a positive development in that it is helpful to have new ideas and insights, but if too many staff members leave, this will cause great disruption and a loss of memory about the initiative.

What can be done to ensure that an initiative continues to improve and be sustained?

This may all seem somewhat bleak, but the good news is that all the necessary tools and frameworks are contained within the building blocks with which you will now be familiar (see Figure 1, in the Preface). As discussed earlier, these are not one-off events to be completed and moved on from, but rather a dynamic set of interactions that must be returned to and repeated throughout the life of an initiative. Therefore, whilst the framework does not provide the answers, it will act as a prompt of the key components that need to be kept in mind as you seek to further improve in the future.

Below we suggest approaches that we have already discussed that would help address the issues outlined above. Note, though, that these are for illustration purposes only, and each situation will, of course, provide its own opportunities and supports.

Keeping your focus

- Regularly review your stakeholder mapping, and ensure that you have regular communication with stakeholders with interest and power (pages 104–106).

- Involve service users and cares in the redesign of pathways to enable co-production and to foster shared ownership (pages 65–77).

- Ensure that your governance and programme board are updated to include changes in the local system (pages 192–197).

- Share findings from evaluative reviews through web-based material and social media along with participation in local good practice and stakeholder events (pages 133–136).

Maintaining your relevance

- Review the initial mapping to test out original assumptions through the use of 'powerful' questions and the 'five whys' to explore less successful processes (pages 48–49 and 37).

- Introduce a survey of key stakeholder representatives to gather in views of what is important and opportunities for improvement at regular intervals (pages 126–127).

- Develop local indicators and data based around the person-centred narrative of integrated care (page 75).

- Draw on reflective debriefing approaches to learn from what has gone well, as well as examples of less positive practice (page 94).

- Collaborate with advocacy and representative groups to undertake 'experts by experience' reviews (pages 67–68).

- Introduce patient held records (PHRs) to give service users more power over their information and to facilitate horizontal data sharing with other services (page 191).

Sustaining your leadership

- Use Appreciative Inquiry (AI) to understand the perspectives of 'followers' as well as 'leaders', and to build on the positives (pages 49–50).

- Be aware of the boundary-spanning roles that you undertake and how you can best gain support from followers across these boundaries (pages 78–83).

- Develop communities of practice with those in leadership roles in other integrated care initiatives, and use leadership frameworks to encourage reflection (pages 107–109 and Chapter 4).

- Develop leaders from all practitioner and professional groups through mentoring and group reflection (page 93).

Strengthening your engagement

- Hold Open Space events with service users, carers, staff and stakeholders to uncover new priorities and opportunities (page 49).

- Review your engagement strategy using the CLEAR framework (pages 64–65).

- Foster a 'culture of enquiry' that includes practitioner-led research and the sharing of findings outside of the discipline and team (page 120).

- Develop inter-professional training that is based around the experiences of service users and includes their direct participation (pages 168–172).

Managing your resources

- Identify the most resource-intensive processes and undertake value stream mapping to strip out any waste (pages 35–36).

- Train staff members in restorative supervision techniques to encourage the sharing of anxiety and developing resistance (pages 90–92).

- Translate performance systems that consider financial and quality aspects into accessible dashboards (pages 192–196).

- Work with the economic departments of local universities to develop cost-effectiveness elements to evaluative reviews (pages 116–118).

- Develop care planning processes that support the development of social networks and other community assets and promote the option of personal budgets (pages 144–146 and pages 155–156).

How is it best to ensure that the end of an initiative is not the end of integrated care?

If an integrated care initiative is starting to address the 'wicked issue' concerned and showing signs of achieving the 'triple aims', then it is to be hoped that investment and support will continue into the long term. An initiative, though, sits within a wider financial, economic and policy context within both its local area and also on a national basis. Senior decision-makers at these levels have to consider multiple and complex issues when reviewing how best to respond to the predicted needs and key opportunities. Subsequent major changes in strategy may result in an integrated care initiative no longer fitting in with the expected structure and partnering arrangements. On a less dramatic basis there may be changes in the roles and responsibilities of other services that then take on much of the work of an integrated care initiative or make it less necessary. In these circumstances, the initiative may gradually feel a bit out of place, with a slow decrease in support and profile rather than a clear decision being made.

These changes in context may be positive in that they could have the capacity and reach to make a considerable impact on a wider population or to address another set of wicked issues. However, this may not be the case, and the new arrangements could have the potential to disrupt but not add. For those who have invested much energy and time into establishing and running an integrated care initiative, this will be a considerable loss and frustration. And there will be rational elements to such feelings – the initiative is now making a difference, there has been considerable investment of staff and other resources, there will be disruption for service users and their carers, and good practice and hard-earned learning may be disregarded. There will also be more emotional and personal reactions related to numerous losses that may be connected with the dismantling of an initiative – a team of colleagues that one believes and trusts in, the fellowship of being part of an aspired vision, and the opportunity to pursue more innovative practice. Such changes can also enable those who doubted that an integrated initiative would succeed to share again their initial concerns and disagreement.

Whilst some of the negative impacts caused by the ending of a service may not be avoidable, it is still possible to positively influence much of the transition process. Such transitions are not often recorded in research or guidance, as we tend to be better at setting out initial hopes and successes than sharing how we coped with an unexpected and unwelcome ending. This is partly because few of us like to publically share our disappointments, but also because, on a practical basis, those involved will have moved on to other roles and responsibilities.

We would suggest that there are three key transitions within the 'ending' of an integrated care initiative that should be considered: *transitions for service users and carers, transitions for professionals and practitioners*, and *transitions of learning*. Using the scenarios that have been developed throughout the book and which were assessed as needing an integrated care initiative, we suggest below how positive transitions could be achieved for integrated care initiatives that did not end as originally planned. Whilst some aspects of these endings could feel like failure for the organisation, for the partnership or for the individual members of staff, we hope that these highlight that it is possible to maintain the pace of change and to sustain the vital drive to better integrated care.

Homeless service

The contract for the homeless service was originally for three years, but was then extended for a further two pending a review of supported housing provision in the locality. During the extension period the local authority commissioner funded an external review of the service. This identified that the hostel was successfully accepting people with complex needs who were unable to access other options due to their behaviour. For those accepted, their quality of life was generally improved, and most had been able to receive support from the relevant health and social care specialist teams. The hostel was able to evidence progression in service users' wellbeing through the regular person-centred reviews that they undertook with engagement from external professionals. They were less aware of what happened to service users following their departure from the hostel, and it was agreed by all the agencies on their steering group to prioritise this for future development.

On the basis of this review the housing association was feeling confident about the potential of winning the contract again. However, the local authority decided to re-tender this service along with a suite of other homeless provision with the hope that a single organisation would deliver them all, and so better integrate their different offers. The housing association delivering this hostel was relatively small and lost the tender to a larger provider with more experience of general homeless services. They were very disappointed not to have the opportunity to further develop the service, but were determined to ensure that the good practice and quality of life of the current tenants were maintained. Meetings were arranged with the new provider as soon as was possible in order to explain the current ethos and approach. Staff members were informed that they would be transferring to the new provider, and were given full details of what this would mean practically for them. They were also given the opportunity to share their emotional reaction. The current tenants were also informed and had individual reviews with their key workers to enable them to discuss any concerns. The current staff team and tenants planned a celebration event, with representatives from the new provider and external agencies also in attendance. A short video was made with the support of a local social enterprise, setting out the story of the hostel and the key lessons that had been learned over the previous five years. The final handover of the service was managed in a relatively smooth and non-confrontational process.

Community rehabilitation service

The service was able to bring together different practitioners and professionals into local teams of nurses, therapists and social workers. These were aligned around groups of general practices, and the local authority reablement service was also restructured so that it worked in similar localities. Clear pathways were put in place regarding hospital avoidance and discharge, and this included the intermediary care beds and befriending scheme run by the voluntary sector. Each locality had a team manager, and these individuals were drawn from a range of disciplines, with an overall service lead. The local authority and health trust provided funding for the management of the service in a pooled budget. Due to the interest on reductions in hospital readmissions and delayed discharges, the service worked with the performance team to develop local measures of their contribution to these processes. They also worked with a local patient representative group to consult with service users about what was important to them, and developed a short questionnaire that could be used with each person to gather their experiences. Along with regular reflective sessions with their staff members, this combined data helped them to identify what was working well and what could be improved. The service was the subject of an external inspection that highlighted a number of areas of excellent practice, and as a result it was flagged up nationally as an exemplar of such working.

General financial pressures led the local authority to review its overall structure in order to make significant savings. There were also concerns about fragmentation between different adult social work specialisms that led to long debates about who would support service users with multiple needs. The review led to the decision that all social workers would be brought back into generic central teams rather than being placed within multi-disciplinary settings. Funding for the management posts was also withdrawn, which meant that the current structure could not be maintained. The service lobbied for an exception to be made in their case, and provided considerable data highlighting the positive impact that they had made in relation to adult social care outcomes and resource usage, and the broader 'triple aims'. However, it was felt that no exceptions could be made, and the social workers were withdrawn. The service lead accepted that they would have to change their integration processes, and therefore started working with the local authority to develop care pathways that would reflect the new arrangements. To ensure that the current workforce could maintain their links and to provide an opportunity for other staff to develop such relationships, it was agreed that joint training opportunities would be provided. Peer networks were also created in relation to particular conditions and issues, with members drawn from across agencies and sectors. A small budget was secured for these networks in order to provide administrative support. Finally, a pattern of six-monthly Open Space events was created in which patient representative groups would meet with staff from the service, the social work teams and other stakeholders to reflect on current experiences and opportunities to improve.

Diabetes service

The arrangements with the diabetes specialists from the hospital were successfully introduced. The GPs with less confidence in supporting patients with diabetes undertook fortnightly reviews with the consultants for those whose condition was worsening. As a consequence, these GPs developed more confidence, and less people needed to be referred to the hospital for treatment. The monthly case discussions involved advanced nurse practitioners from the diabetes team, and this enabled a multi-disciplinary discussion that was informative to all concerned. The practice nurses initially found their role in health promotion difficult due to their other demands, and as many of them were from a different cultural background to the patients, they sometimes struggled to identify relevant and appropriate alternative options. However, a grant was obtained to provide additional capacity in the practice nurse team, and this also enabled training regarding the cultural aspects. This included spending time with local community groups, which all of them enjoyed. The voluntary sector group was able to recruit to its physical activity worker post. They linked up with local leisure centres to promote current fitness opportunities, and following feedback from the community, also developed women-only sessions.

The diabetes service was led by one of the local GPs with a particular interest in this condition working closely with a practice nurse and the consultant from the acute hospital. The GP was offered a post at a local university, in part because of her work in relation to this initiative, and the practice nurse had to move to another area due to family circumstances. They initially tried to find other practice members to take on these lead roles, but there were none who had the confidence or interest in doing so. They therefore decided to look again at what was needed, and worked with the wider practice teams, voluntary sector group and the secondary service to undertake an evaluative review of what was needed. This process highlighted that the health promotion activities were now embedded in the work of the practice nurses, and the GPs were much more competent in diagnosing and treating service users with diabetes. The voluntary sector group had managed to develop a social enterprise that would generate sufficient funding to be self-sustainable through selling wellbeing advice to surrounding areas. It was therefore decided that the initial structure of meetings and reviews was no longer required. This was replaced by a network arrangement in which the interested stakeholders would meet every quarter to share experiences and gain others' views on current challenges. This would be coordinated by the diabetes consultant's secretary. There was also an ongoing opportunity for the general practice staff to contact the diabetes service whenever they wanted guidance, and for surveys to be given to patients every six months. The first article that the new academic GP wrote was based on the service, and the organisations collectively submitted a bid for a national award.

Conclusion

As set out in the Preface, integrated care is not a fixed thing but instead is a fluid state that requires constant amending and adapting. Each individual and their social, health and housing situation are unique, and the package of support and the connections that they require are also unique. Services, organisations and policy frameworks under which professionals and practitioners operate will change over time. In some cases this will be a radical change in which an organisation or service is no longer in existence or dramatically reconfigured, whereas for others it will be more incremental and there will be steady changes over time. The wider economic and technological environment is also constantly changing, with new challenges and opportunities being presented as a consequence. All these changes have the potential to result in new, emerging fragmentations as existing patterns and routines are disrupted and as relationships between key individuals no longer become central to processes and systems. Such change also provides the opportunity for doing things differently and building in improvements in how services work together within new models and approaches. Integrated care is, then, a long-term endeavour which will never be 'sorted' as such, but which will always require our attention and energies.

In this book we have attempted to share current academic and practice knowledge of what works in integration to support those who are leading the integration in practice. Reflecting the field as a whole, developments such as these are in many ways out of date the moment they are written, and this is particularly the case in such an exciting time of integrated care. However, the principles, and the thinking that lies behind them, do last beyond a particular initiative or problem. It is our belief and experience that grasping, understanding and applying the various tools and approaches that have been outlined will provide a toolkit of knowledge and understanding which will enable integrated care leaders to respond to what may lie ahead. We hope this will assist in creating a vision in which service users and carers can expect their needs to be recognised, their views to be listened to and for their lives to be enriched through collaboration between a diverse range of practitioners and professions. We would genuinely welcome any feedback on what is helpful and what could be improved, as well as your examples of learning that you think could be shared in future editions.

References

Atkinson, M., Jones, M. and Lamont, E. (2007) *Multi-agency Working and its Implications for Practice.* Reading: CfBT Education Trust.

Bandura, A. (1995) *Self-efficacy in Changing Societies.* Cambridge: Cambridge University Press.

Barlow, J., Wright, C., Sheasby, J., Turner, A. and Hainsworth, A. (2002) 'Self-management approaches for people with chronic conditions: a review.' *Patient Education and Counseling 48,* 2, 177–187.

Barr, H. (1998) 'Competent to collaborate: towards a competency-based model for interprofessional education.' *Journal of Interprofessional Care 12,* 2, 181–187.

Bate, P. and Robert, G. (2006) 'Experience-based design: from redesigning the system around the patient to co-designing services with the patient.' *Quality & Safety in Health Care 15,* 5, October, 307–310.

Berwick, D. M., Nolan, T. W. and Whittington, J. (2008) 'The triple aim: care, health, and cost.' *Health Affairs 27,* 3, 759–769.

Better Care Fund (2015) *How to Understand and Measure Impact.* Available at http://www.scie.org.uk/health-social-integrated-care/better-care/implementation-support/how-to-understand-and-measure-impact.pdf, accessed on 12 May 2016.

Bowers, H., Bailey, G., Sanderson, H., Bown, H., Easterbrook, L. and Macadam, A. (2007) *Person-centred Thinking with Older People: Practicalities and Possibilities.* Stockport: Helen Sanderson Associates Press.

Cameron, A., Lart, R., Bostock, L. and Coomber, C. (2012) *Factors that Promote and Hinder Joint and Integrated Working Between Health and Social Care Services.* Available at www.scie.org.uk, accessed on 7 December 2015.

Carpenter, J., Webb, C., Bostock, L. and Coomber, C. (2012) *Effective Supervision in Social Work and Social Care.* Available at www.scie.org.uk/publications/briefings/files/briefing43.pdf, accessed on 7 December 2015.

Cornes, M., Manthorpe, J., Hennessy, C., Anderson, S., Clark, M. and Scanlon, C. (2014) 'Not just a talking shop: practitioner perspectives on how communities of practice work to improve outcomes for people experiencing multiple exclusion homelessness.' *Journal of Interprofessional Care 28,* 6, 541–546.

D'Amour, D. and Oandasan, I. (2005) 'Interprofessionality as the field of interprofessional practice and interprofessional education: an emerging concept.' *Journal of Interprofessional Care 19,* S1, 8–20.

DH (Department of Health) (2005) *Self Care – A Real Choice.* London: DH.

Ellins, J., Glasby, J., Tanner, D., McIver, S., *et al.* (2012) *Understanding and Improving Transitions of Older People: A User and Carer Centred Approach.* London: The National Institute for Health Research.

Ernst, C. and Chrobot-Mason, D. (2010) *Boundary Spanning Leadership: Six Practices for Solving Problems, Driving Innovation, and Transforming Organizations.* New York: McGraw Hill Professional.

Ernst, C. and Yip, J. (2009) 'Boundary Spanning Leadership: Tactics to Bridge Social Identity Groups in Organizations.' In T. Pittinsky (ed.) *Crossing the Divide: Intergroup Leadership in a World of Difference.* Boston, MA: Harvard Business School Press.

Ferlie, E. B. and Shortell, S. M. (2001) 'Improving the quality of health care in the United Kingdom and the United States: a framework for change.' *Milbank Quarterly 79,* 2, 281–315.

Frontier Economics (2012) *Enablers and Barriers to Integrated Care and Implications for Monitor.* Available at https://www.gov.uk/guidance/enabling-integrated-care-in-the-nhs, accessed on 7 December 2015.

Fulop, N., Mowlem, A. and Edwards, N. (2005) *Building Integrated Care: Lessons from the UK and Elsewhere.* London: The NHS Confederation.

Galdas, P., Darwin, Z., Kidd, L., Blickem, C., *et al.* (2014) 'The accessibility and acceptability of self-management support interventions for men with long term conditions: a systematic review and meta-synthesis of qualitative studies.' *BMC Public Health 14,* 1230.

Gale, N. K., Shapiro, J., McLeod, H. S., Redwood, S. and Hewison, A. (2014) 'Patients–people–place: developing a framework for researching organizational culture during health service redesign and change.' *Implementation Science 9,* 1, 106.

Gamiz, R. and Tsegai, A. (2014) 'Beyond practitioner-research: integration to outcomes.' *Journal of Integrated Care 22,* 3, 108–116.

Gibbs, G. (1988) *Learning by Doing: A Guide to Teaching and Learning Methods.* Oxford: Further Education Unit, Oxford Brookes University.

Glasby, J. (2005) 'The integration dilemma: how deep and how broad to go?' *Journal of Integrated Care 13,* 5, 27–30.

Glasby, J., Miller, R. and Posaner, R. (2013) *New Conversations Between Old Players? The Relationship Between General Practice and Social Care in an Era of Clinical Commissioning.* London: School for Social Care Research.

Goleman, D. (2000) 'Leadership that gets results.' *Harvard Business Review,* March–April.

Grint, K. and Holt, C. (2011) *Followership in the NHS: Commission on Leadership and Management in the NHS.* London: King's Fund.

Hardy, B., Hudson, B. and Waddington, E. (2003) *Assessing Strategic Partnership: The Partnership Assessment Tool.* London: Office of the Deputy Prime Minister. Available at http://webarchive.nationalarchives.gov.uk/20120919132719/http://www.communities.gov.uk/documents/localgovernment/pdf/135112.pdf, accessed on 7 December 2015.

Harris, R., Sims, S., Hewitt, G., Joy, M., *et al.* (2013) *Interprofessional Teamwork Across Stroke Care Pathways: Outcomes and Patient and Carer Experience. Final Report.* NIHR Service Delivery and Organisation Programme. London: National Institute for Health Research.

Health Foundation, The (2014) *Spreading Improvement Ideas: Tips from Empirical Research. Evidence Scan No. 20.* London: The Health Foundation.

Heifetz, R. (1994) *Leadership without Easy Answers.* Cambridge: Harvard University Press.

Heifetz, R. A. and Linsky, M. (2002) 'A survival guide for leaders.' *Harvard Business Review 80,* 6, 65–74.

Heifetz, R., Grashow, A., and Linsky, M. (2009) *The Practice of Adaptive Leadership.* Boston, MA: Harvard Business School Publishing.

Hersey, P. and Blanchard, K. H. (1969) *Management of Organizational Behavior.* Englewood Cliffs, NJ: Prentice-Hall,

Hibbard, J. H., Stockard, J., Mahoney, E. R. and Tusler, M. (2004) 'Development of the Patient Activation Measure (PAM): conceptualizing and measuring activation in patients and consumers.' *Health Services Research 39,* 4.1, 1005–1026.

Iles, V. and Sutherland, K. (2001) *Managing Change in the NHS. Organisational Change: A Review for Health Care Managers, Professionals and Researchers.* London: National Coordinating Centre for NHS Service Delivery and Organisation R&D.

Inter-professional Education Collaborative Expert Panel (2011) *Core Competencies for Inter-professional Collaborative Practice: Report of an Expert Panel.* Washington, DC: Inter-professional Education Collaborative.

Jelphs, K., Dickinson, H. and Miller, R. (2016) *Working in Teams.* Bristol: Policy Press.

Jenkins, L., Brigden, C. and King, A. (2013) 'Evaluating a third sector community service following stroke.' *Journal of Integrated Care 21,* 5, 248–262.

Johnson, G. and Scholes, K. (2001) *Exploring Corporate Strategy.* 6th edn. Upper Saddle River, NJ: Prentice Hall.

Kelly, J. (2015) 'Integrating occupational therapy services – playing the long game.' *Journal of Integrated Care 23,* 4, 185–193.

Kennedy, A., Reeves, D., Bower, P., Lee, V., *et al.* (2007) 'The effectiveness and cost effectiveness of a national lay-led self care support programme for patients with long-term conditions: a pragmatic randomised controlled trial.' *Journal of Epidemiology and Community Health 61*, 3, March, 254–261.

Kirkpatrick, D. L. and Kirkpatrick, J. D. (2007) *Implementing the Four Levels.* San Francisco, CA: Berrett-Koehler Publishers Inc.

Kislov, R., Walshe, K. and Harvey, G. (2012) 'Managing boundaries in primary care service improvement: a developmental approach to communities of practice.' *Implementation Science 7*, 1, 97.

Kodner, D. L. and Spreeuwenberg, C. (2002) 'Integrated care: meaning, logic, applications, and implications – a discussion paper.' *International Journal of Integrated Care 2.* Available at http://www.ncbi.nlm.nih.gov/pmc/articles/PMC1480401, accessed on 16 May 2016.

Kotter, J. (1990) *A Force for Change – How Leadership Differs from Management.* New York: Free Press.

Kotter, J. (1996) *Leading Change.* Boston, MA: Harvard Business School Press.

Leadership for Change programme, Safe-fail experiments handout produced for Residential session 1, 2014. Available at http://leadershipforchange.org.uk/learning-centre/residential-1-materials, accessed on 7 December 2015.

Leutz, W. N. (1999) 'Five laws for integrating medical and social services: lessons from the United States and the United Kingdom.' *Milbank Quarterly 77*, 1, 77–110.

Löffler, E. (2010) *Why Co-production is an Important Topic for Local Government: Local Authorities Research Council Initiative (LARCI).* Governance International. Available at www.govint.org/fileadmin/user_upload/publications/coproduction_why_it_is_important.pdf, accessed on 13 January 2016.

Lowndes, V., Pratchett, P. and Stoker, G. (2006) 'Diagnosing and remedying the failings of official participation schemes: the CLEAR framework.' *Social Policy and Society 5*, 281–291.

Magnezi, R., Bergman, Y. S. and Grosberg, D. (2014) 'Online activity and participation in treatment affects the perceived efficacy of social health networks among patients with chronic illness.' *Journal of Medical Internet Research 16*, 1, e12.

Matland, R. E. (1995) 'Synthesizing the implementation literature: the ambiguity-conflict model of policy implementation.' *Journal of Public Administration Research and Theory 5*, 2, 145–174.

Miller, R. (2013) *Is Integration or Fragmentation the Starting Point to Improve Prevention?* Birmingham: Health Services Management Centre, University of Birmingham. Available at www.birmingham.ac.uk/Documents/college-social-sciences/social-policy/HSMC/publications/PolicyPapers/policy-paper-seventeen.pdf, accessed on 7 December 2015.

Miller, R., Combes, G., Brown, H. and Harwood, A. (2014) 'Interprofessional workplace learning: a catalyst for strategic change?' *Journal of Interprofessional Care 28*, 3, 186–193.

Miller, R., Freeman, T., Davidson, D. and Glasby, J. (2015) *An Adult Social Care Compendium of Approaches and Tools for Organisational Change.* Birmingham and London: Health Services Management Centre, University of Birmingham; Middlesex University. Available at www.birmingham.ac.uk/Documents/college-social-sciences/social-policy/HSMC/publications/change-compendium-2015.pdf, accessed on 14 January 2016.

Miller, S. M. (1987) 'Monitoring and blunting: validation of a questionnaire to assess styles of information seeking under threat.' *Journal of Personality and Social Psychology 52*, 2, February, 345–353. Available at http://dx.doi.org/10.1037/0022-3514.52.2.345, accessed on 13 January 2016.

Minkman, M. N., Ahaus, K. T. B. and Huijsman, R. (2009) 'A four phase development model for integrated care services in the Netherlands.' *BMC Health Services Research 9*, 42. Available at www.ncbi.nlm.nih.gov/pmc/articles/PMC2660899, accessed on 13 January 2016.

National Voices (2013) *A Narrative for Person-centred Coordinated Care.* Available at www.england.nhs.uk/wp-content/uploads/2013/05/nv-narrative-cc.pdf, accessed on 17 November 2015.

NHS England (2015) *Using Case Finding and Risk Stratification: A Key Service Component for Personalised Care and Support Planning.* Available at https://www.england.nhs.uk/wp-content/uploads/2015/01/2015-01-20-CFRS-v0.14-FINAL.pdf, accessed on 31 March 2016.

Nolte, E. and Pitchforth, E. (2014) *What is the Evidence on the Economic Impacts of Integrated Care?* Denmark: World Health Organization.

Ogrinc, G., Davies, L., Goodman, D., Batalden, P., Davidoff, F. and Stevens, D. (2015) 'SQUIRE 2.0 (Standards for QUality Improvement Reporting Excellence): revised publication guidelines from a detailed consensus process.' *The Journal of Continuing Education in Nursing 46*, 11, 501–507.

OPM (2015) *Evaluation of the Leading Integrated System Level Change Programme: Report to the Advancing Quality Alliance (AQuA)*. Available at www.opm.co.uk/publications/evaluation-of-aquas-leading-integrated-system-level-change-programme, accessed on 28 November 2015.

Pardo del Val, M. and Martinez, C. (2003) 'Resistance to change: a literature review and empirical study.' *Management Decision 41*, 2, 148–155.

Petch, A. (2012) 'Tectonic plates: aligning evidence, policy and practice in health and social care integration.' *Journal of Integrated Care 20*, 2, 77–88.

Piette, J. D., Resnicow, K., Choi, H. and Heisler, M. (2013) 'A diabetes peer support intervention that improved glycemic control: mediators and moderators of intervention effectiveness.' *Chronic Illness 9*, 4, December.

Quenk, N. L. (1996) *In the Grip: Our Hidden Personality*. Palo Alto, CA: Consulting Psychologists Press.

RAND Europe (2012) *National Evaluation of DH Integrated Care Pilots*. Available at www.gov.uk/government/publications/national-evaluation-of-department-of-healths-integrated-care-pilots, accessed on 7 December 2015.

Reeves, D., Blickem, C., Vassilev, I., Brooks, H., *et al.* (2014) 'The contribution of social networks to the health and self-management of patients with long-term conditions: a longitudinal study.' *PLoS ONE 9*, 6, e98340.

Robson, C. (2002) *Real World Research: A Resource for Social Scientists and Practitioner-Researchers* (Vol. 2). Oxford: Blackwell.

Rogers, A., Vassilev, I., Kennedy, A., Blickem, C., Reeves, D. and Brooks, H. (2014) 'Why less may be more? A mixed methods study of the work and relatedness of "weak" ties in supporting long term condition self-management.' *Implementation Science 9*, 19.

Rogers, E. (2003) *Diffusion of Innovations*. 5th edn. New York: Free Press.

Rummery, K. (2009) 'Healthy partnerships, healthy citizens? An international review of partnerships in health and social care and patient/user outcomes.' *Social Science & Medicine 69*, 1797–1804.

Sanderson, H. and Miller, R. (2014) *The Individual Service Funds Handbook: Implementing Personal Budgets in Provider Organisations*. London: Jessica Kingsley Publishers.

Schein, E. H. (2010) *Organizational Culture and Leadership*, Vol. 2. Chichester: John Wiley & Sons.

SCIE (Social Care Institute for Excellence) (2013) *Effective Supervision in a Variety of Settings*. London: SCIE.

Stacey, R. D. (2009) *Complexity and Organizational Reality, Uncertainty and the Need to Rethink Management after the Collapse of Investment Capitalism*. 2nd edn. London: Routledge.

Steventon, A., Bardsley, M., Billings, J., Georghiou, T. and Lewis, G. (2011) *An Evaluation of the Impact of Community-based Services on Hospital Usage*. London: Nuffield Trust.

Tucker, H. and Burgis, M. (2012) 'Patients set the agenda on integrating community services in Norfolk.' *Journal of Integrated Care 20*, 4, 231–240.

Vangen, S., Hayes, J. P. and Cornforth, C. (2015) 'Governing cross-sector, inter-organizational collaborations.' *Public Management Review 17*, 9, 1237–1260.

Vassilev, I., Rogers, A., Blickem, C., Brooks, H., *et al.* (2013) 'Social networks, and the "work" and work force of chronic illness self-management: a survey analysis of personal communities.' *PloS ONE 8*, e59723.

Vassilev, I., Rogers, A., Kennedy, A. and Koetsenruijter, J. (2014) 'The influence of social networks on self-management support: a metasynthesis.' *BMC Public Health 14*, 719.

Walker, G. and Gillies, L. (2014) '"Sliding Doors": innovative approaches to supporting culture change.' *Journal of Integrated Care 22*, 4, 154–164. Available at www.knowledge.scot.nhs.uk/home/portals-and-topics/care-for-older-people-portal/reshaping-care-for-older-people/sliding-doors-learning-resource.aspx, accessed on 13 January 2016.

Wallbank, S. (2011) 'Restorative supervision manual.' *NHS Midlands and East Restorative Clinical Supervision Programme 44*, 4.18, 42–81.

Weick, K. E. and Quinn, R. E. (1999) 'Organizational change and development.' *Annual Review of Psychology 50*, 361–386.

Weir, B. and Fillingham, D. (2014) *System Leadership, Lessons and Learning from AQuA's Integrated Care Discovery Communities*. London: King's Fund.

Wenger, E., McDermott, R. and Snyder, W. M. (2002) *Cultivating Communities of Practice.* Boston, MA: Harvard Business School Press.

West, M. A. and Lyubovnikova, J. (2013) 'Illusions of team working in health care.' *Journal of Health Organization and Management 27*, 1, 134–142.

Woolham, J. (2011) *Research Governance and Ethics for Adult Social Care Research: Procedures, Practices and Challenges.* London: London School of Economics and Political Science.

Resources

Organisations (general)
European Observatory on Health Systems and Policies

www.euro.who.int/en/about-us/partners/observatory

Supports and promotes evidence-based health policy-making through comprehensive and rigorous analysis of the dynamics of healthcare systems in Europe. Its website includes news items, policy briefs and summaries, and the BRIDGE series of key lessons and best practice to inform health policy-makers and to foster evidence into practice.

The Health Foundation

www.health.org.uk

An independent charity committed to bringing about better health and healthcare for people in the UK through its programme of commissioned research.

Health Services Management Centre (HSMC) at the University of Birmingham

www.birmingham.ac.uk/schools/social-policy/departments/
health-services-management-centre/index.aspx

One of the leading centres in the UK for the provision of research, teaching, professional development and consultancy to health and social care agencies. For more than 40 years, HSMC has been conducting high-quality, original, policy-relevant research into the organisation, coordination and effectiveness of health and social care services, and helps to shape policy and practice in the UK and abroad.

Institute for Healthcare Improvement (IHI)

www.ihi.org

An independent not-for-profit organisation based in the US. For more than 25 years it has been a leading innovator, convener, partner and driver of results in health and healthcare improvement worldwide.

Institute of Local Government Studies (INLOGOV) at the University of Birmingham

www.birmingham.ac.uk/schools/government-society/
departments/local-government-studies/index.aspx

The leading academic centre for research and teaching on local governance and strategic public management. With over 40 years' experience working within local government and the public sector, INLOGOV creates the latest thinking for public servants.

Institute for Research and Innovation in Social Services (Iriss)

www.iriss.org.uk

A charitable company working to enhance the capacity and capability of the social services workforce in Scotland by enabling access to, and promoting the use of, knowledge and research for service innovation and improvement.

International Federation for Integrated Care (IFIC)

http://integratedcarefoundation.org

A not-for-profit educational membership-based network that crosses organisational and professional boundaries in order to bring people together to advance the science, knowledge and adoption of integrated care policy and practice.

The King's Fund

www.kingsfund.org.uk

An independent charity working to improve health and healthcare in England. It helps shape policy and practice through research and analysis; develops individuals, teams and organisations; promotes understanding of the health and social care system; and brings people together to learn, share knowledge and debate. Its online resources also include video clips of key speakers leading UK and international integrated care projects: www.kingsfund.org.uk/topics/integrated-care.

Leadership Centre

www.localleadership.gov.uk

Created and launched in 2004, this organisation acquired charitable status as the Leadership Centre for Local Government in April 2008. It works closely with the Local Government Association (see below) to support, promote and improve local government.

Local Government Association

www.local.gov.uk

A politically led, cross-party membership organisation that works on behalf of councils to ensure local government has a strong, credible voice with national government. The organisation aims to influence and set the political agenda on the issues that matter to councils so they are able to deliver local solutions to national problems.

National Institute for Health and Care Excellence (NICE)

www.evidence.nhs.uk

Provides national guidance, advice and evidence-based recommendations on a wide range of topics, from preventing and managing specific conditions, to providing social care to adults and children, and planning broader services and interventions to improve the health of communities. These aim to promote integrated care where appropriate, for example by covering transitions between children's and adult services and between health and social care.

National Voices

www.nationalvoices.org.uk

Brings the voices of patients, service users and carers to bear on national health and social care policy in England. The organisation works with its membership to influence government ministers and departments, professional bodies and other organisations, and to ensure that policy focuses on delivering what matters most to patients and service users and their families and carers.

Nesta (National Endowment for Science Technology and the Arts)

www.nesta.org.uk

An independent charity dedicated to supporting ideas that can help improve lives, with activities ranging from early stage investment to in-depth research and practical programmes. Its areas of work include health and ageing and citizen engagement in public services. The Centre for Social Action Innovation Fund is a partnership between Nesta and the Cabinet Office, with funds being provided to support a range of activities and projects with a strong engagement focus.

Nuffield Trust

www.nuffieldtrust.org.uk

An independent health charity that aims to improve the quality of healthcare in the UK by providing evidence-based research and policy analysis and informing and generating debate.

Royal College of General Practitioners (RCGP)

www.rcgp.org.uk/policy/rcgp-policy-areas/integration-of-care.aspx

Has long championed the development of integrated care, and this web page collects together some of the work the organisation has done in this area, including their policy paper on integrated care published in 2012.

Social Care Institute for Excellence (SCIE)

www.scie.org.uk

A leading improvement support agency and independent charity, working with the care and support sector in the UK. The organisation co-produces its work with people who use services and carers.

Virtual Staff College

www.virtualstaffcollege.co.uk

Designs and delivers professional development opportunities for leaders in local authority children's services and other stakeholders such as health and wellbeing boards, clinical commissioning groups and other partners, working in services for children, young people and families.

World Health Organization (WHO)

www.who.int/servicedeliverysafety/areas/people-centred-care/en

Created in 1948 with the primary role of directing and coordinating international health within the United Nations' system. The organisation's global strategy on people-centred and integrated health services represents a call for a fundamental shift in the way health services are funded, managed and delivered. The strategy is made up of two linked documents – the first of which is the strategy itself, whilst the second is an overview of good practice, which presents a number of case studies and the evidence on the benefits that people-centred and integrated care can bring to people, communities and countries.

Organisations (advocacy)
Age UK

www.ageuk.org.uk

Other charities for specific conditions/diseases are also useful, e.g. Diabetes UK.

Gov.uk

https://www.gov.uk/government/collections/mental-capacity-act-making-decisions

Provides information for making decisions under the Mental Capacity Act.

Mencap

https://www.mencap.org.uk/our-services/personal-support-services/advocacy/empower-me

Mencap is the voice of learning disability.

NHS Choices

www.nhs.uk/conditions/social-care-and-support-guide/pages/advocacy-services.aspx

Provides information on advocacy services.

Older People's Advocacy Alliance (OPAAL)

www.opaal.org.uk

Advocacy for older people.

Social Care Institute for Excellence (SCIE)

www.scie.org.uk/independent-mental-health-advocacy

Provides information on Independent Mental Health Advocacy.

Journals

Health & Social Care in the Community

http://onlinelibrary.wiley.com/journal/10.1111/(ISSN)1365-2524

An international peer-reviewed journal with a multi-disciplinary audience.

International Journal of Integrated Care

www.integratedcarefoundation.org

The Integrated Foundation for Integrated Care is an international collaboration that hosts this open-access journal.

Journal of Integrated Care

www.emeraldinsight.com/journal/jica

The UK's leading journal looking at practice, policy and the research of integrated care.

Journal of Interprofessional Care

www.tandfonline.com/action/journalInformation?show=aims Scope&journalCode=ijic20#.VioDGH7nvIU

Aims to disseminate research and new developments in the field of interprofessional education and practice.

Subject Index

Author Index